Residential Choices
and Experiences of
Older Adults

Pathways to Life Quality

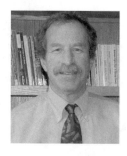 **John A. Krout,** Ph.D., received his doctorate in sociology from Penn State University in 1977 and is Professor of Gerontology and Director of the Gerontology Institute at Ithaca College. He has written some 60 book chapters and articles and published in a wide range of academic journals such as *The Gerontologist, Research on Aging, International Journal of Aging and Human Development*, and *Journal of Gerontology*, and has made some 150 presentations at national and state conferences on rural aging issues and community-based services for older adults. His books include, *The Aged in Rural America, Senior Centers in America, Providing Community-Based Services to the Rural Elderly*, and the recently published *Aging in Rural Settings*, with Raymond T. Coward, as well as several bibliographies on rural aging. He is past-president of the State Society on Aging of New York, a Fellow of the Gerontological Society of America, and a charter fellow of the Association of Gerontology in Higher Education.

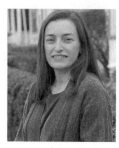 **Elaine Wethington,** Ph.D., is Associate Professor of Human Development and of Sociology at Cornell University, Ithaca and chair of its institutional review board. She is currently serving as Co-Director of the Cornell Gerontology Research Institute. Wethington is a medical sociologist, specializing in the study of stressors and mental health. She received her Ph.D. from the University of Michigan. Wethington is currently conducting a series of national studies on the relationship between recent life events and social integration as well as co-leading the Pathways to Life Quality study. She has also collaborated with other researchers on studies of stressor exposure.

Residential Choices
and Experiences of
Older Adults
Pathways to Life Quality

John A. Krout, PhD
Elaine Wethington, PhD
Editors

 Springer Publishing Company

Copyright © 2003 by Springer Publishing Company, Inc.

All rights reserved

No part of this publication may be reproduced, stored in a retrieval system, or transmitted in any form or by any means, electronic, mechanical, photocopying, recording, or otherwise, without the prior permission of Springer Publishing Company, Inc.

Springer Publishing Company, Inc.
536 Broadway
New York, NY 10012-3955

Acquisitions Editor: Helvi Gold
Production Editor: Janice Stangel
Cover design by Joanne Honigman

01   02   03   04   05 / 5   4   3   2   1

Library of Congress Cataloging-in-Publication Data

Residential choices and experiences of older adults : pathways to life quality /
    John A. Krout, Elaine Wethington, editor.
        p.   cm.
    Includes bibliographical refernces and index.
    ISBN 0-8261-1954-9
    1. Aged—Housing—United States—Decision making.   2. Aged—
Housing—United States—Planning.   3. Quality of Life—Aged—United
States.   I. Title Pathways to life quality.   II. Krout, John A.
III. Wethington, Elaine.

HD7287.92.US4R47 2003
363.5'946'0973—dc21

                                                    2003042788

Printed in the United States of America by Maple-Vail Book Manufacturing Group

Dedication

This book is dedicated to the older adults who graciously shared their time and life experiences as participants in the *Pathways to Life Quality* study.

JAK
EW

CONTENTS

Contributors

Katherine Beissner, PhD, PT, is Professor in the Department of Physical Therapy at Ithaca College. She is a member of the American Physical Therapy Association sections on Research, Orthopedics, Geriatrics and Education, and serves on the board of directors of Ithacare, a senior living facility. Dr. Beissner's research interests include the relationships among physical abilities, functional status, and housing needs for older adults.

Alice Boyce, is Project Manager/Research for the Pathways to Life Quality Study at Cornell University. She has a Master's degree in sociology with a specialization in social gerontology from the Pennsylvania State University. She is a member of the Gerontological Society of America and the New York State Society on Aging. She has participated in research projects on topics such as Alzheimer's caregiving, medical and psychiatric comorbidities, ethnic differences in religiosity and spirituality and the effects on well-being, promotion of cancer screening for older women, environmental modifications, and intergenerational relationships.

Donna Dempster-McClain received a Ph.D. from Cornell University in Human Development and Family Studies and is Associate Director of the Bronfenbrenner Life Course Center and Senior Lecturer in the Department of Human Development at Cornell University from 1992–2002. Her research and teaching interests focus on social gerontology and life course transitions. She served as the Project Director for the Cornell Women's Roles and Well-Being Study from 1985–1992 and was an Associate Professor of Child and Family Development at California State University Long Beach, from 1970–1983.

Mary Ann Erickson is Assistant Professor in the Ithaca College Gerontology Institute. Her research focuses on volunteering and social integration among older adults. She has a Ph.D. in Human Development from Cornell University, and is a member of the Gerontological Society of America and the State Society on Aging of New York.

Paul E. Eshelman is Associate Professor in the Department of Design and Environmental Analysis at Cornell University. He has a Masters of Fine Arts Degree from the University of Illinois in industrial design. Before coming to Cornell, he designed train interiors for Amtrak in Washington, DC, and furniture for Herman Miller Research Corporation, Ann Arbor, Michigan. At Cornell, he teaches interior and furniture design. He is a past Editor of the *Journal of Interior Design*, a refereed journal published by the Interior Design Educators Council. His research interest is design for special populations with an emphasis on older adults, especially people with Alzheimer's disease.

Gary W. Evans received his Ph.D. from the University of Massachusetts-Amherst and is professor of design and environmental analysis and of human development at Cornell

University. His primary scholarly interests include environmental stress, children's environments, and poverty.

Heidi H. Holmes was the Project Manager/Director of Data Collections for the Pathways to Life Quality Study in the Gerontology Institute of Ithaca College from 1999–2002. She previously was Research Coordinator at the Children and Family Research Center at the University of Illinois at Urbana-Champaign and Instructor of Psychology at Eastern Illinois University. She holds a Master of Arts degree in experimental psychology/statistics. At present, she is a doctoral student in Gerontology at the University of Kentucky. Her research interests are aging, women's health, stress, and coping. She is a member of the Gerontological Society of America and an associate member of the American Psychological Association.

Phyllis Moen is Ferris Family Professor Life Course Studies and Professor of Sociology and of Human Development at Cornell University, where she is a founding director of the Bronfenbrenner Life Course Center. Her research focuses on gender and aging over the life course, and is funded by the Alfred P. Sloan foundation and the National Institute on Aging. Her latest book is *It's About Time: Couples and Careers*. Other books include *Working Parents, Women's Two Roles*, and, as co-author, *Examining Lives in Context, The State of Americans*, and *A Nation Divided*. Moen received her Ph.D. in Sociology from the University of Minnesota in 1978, and her B.S. and M.A. from the University of North Dakota.

Karl Pillemer is Professor of Human Development at Cornell University, where he directs the Cornell Gerontology Research Institute, one of five Edward R. Roybal Centers on Applied Gerontology established nationwide by the National Institute on Aging. He received a Ph.D. in Sociology from Brandeis University. His interests center on human development over the life course, with a special emphasis on family and social relationships in middle age and beyond. He has conducted major studies on the topic of family caregiving, funded over the past 15 years by the National Institutes of Health. A second research interest is in intergenerational relations in later life, with a focus on determinants and consequences of the quality of adult child-parent relationships. Pillemer is also involved in intervention research on ways of improving nursing home care. He recently co-edited the book *Social Integration in the Second Half of Life*.

Shinobu Utamura was born on November 17, 1976, in Ibaraki, Japan. She came to America to pursue a Master's degree in the area of Housing and Design. She graduated from Cornell University with a M.S. degree in the College of Human Ecology, Department of Design and Environmental Analysis in August, 2001. She works as a usability specialist at Fujitsu Co., Ltd. in Japan. Her research interest is how humans are affected by their environment, and how these elements should be controlled and taken into account in the course of human-centered design. She explores her interest in the field of Universal Design as well as software and web usability.

Kelly Welsh received her M.S. degree in physical therapy from Ithaca College in 2002. She served as president of the Ithaca College Physical Therapy student organization and received the 2002 Ithaca College Physical Therapy Faculty Award. She also was a guest lecturer in gerontology at the 20012 New York American Physical Therapy Association Southern Tier Symposium.

Sarah Wolle holds a B.A. in Psychology and a M.S. in Recreation and Leisure Studies from the State University of New York at Purchase and Cortland respectively. She is a Certified Therapeutic Recreation Specialist. While at Ithaca College, she worked on the Pathways to Life Quality Study as a research assistant and was an instructor in the Therapeutic Recreation and Leisure Services Department. Recently, Sarah became a National Institute of Aging pre-doctoral fellow at The Pennsylvania State University where she is majoring in Leisure Studies and minoring in Gerontology.

Foreword

I was honored to be asked to serve as a member of the National Advisory Board to the Pathways Study because this groundbreaking project addressed an important and looming policy concern for our nation—the role of housing decisions and transitions in determining the life quality of older Americans. Similarly, I am honored to write the forward for this book that represents the cumulative efforts of an impressive interdisciplinary team of researchers who partnered with a diverse group of housing providers and residents over a five-year period to explore this issue.

As a researcher and policymaker, I have struggled for years to highlight the significance of the housing dimension as a factor in quality of care and quality of life outcomes for older adults. Pioneers in environmental psychology and housing design, in particular the late Powell Lawton, worked throughout their careers to emphasize that "where and how people live" are major contributors to the well-being of people as they age. In my 1999 monograph published by the Milbank Memorial Fund, I argued that housing must be considered equally important to the delivery of services and supports in extending the potential for individuals with chronic illness and disabilities to live as independently as possible in the community. The research findings and discussion presented in this book affirm my argument and, furthermore, underscore the complex nature of housing choices and how they interact with life circumstances to determine how older adults fare over time.

This study represents a major contribution to the field of gerontology for several reasons. First, it is one of the few investigations in recent history to explore housing decisions and the implications of moving and relocation across a wide range of residential settings from private homes to small group homes to large assisted living facilities. Second, the diversity of populations studied, including individuals from vastly different socioeconomic backgrounds, provides a valuable opportunity to examine how income and wealth affect housing choices and access to services. This is a key issue for public policy since the majority of activities in housing development have occurred in the private sector for older adults "with the means" to pay for it. Third, the focus on the life course perspective and, in particular, understanding housing decisions and transitions within the context of individuals' life histories, offers important insights into how residential choices are influenced and shaped over time.

The authors must be congratulated for their steadfast commitment to interdisciplinary and intercollegiate research throughout the study. Those of us who have attempted to develop research partnerships know how difficult such an activity can be. The fact that over 125 students and two dozen faculty members participated in the data collection, analysis and dissemination of findings is a testament to the importance of this issue and the tenacity of the project's leadership.

A little over three years ago, I created an Institute within the American Association of Homes and Services for the Aging—an association of non-profit long-term care and housing providers—with the goal of bridging the worlds of research, policy and practice. The study described in this book is an example of just such an enterprise. The research team did not develop their study in an ivory tower. Rather, they used real-world settings as natural laboratories to assess how older adults make housing choices, how relocation affects their quality of life, and how individuals with different levels of physical and cognitive functioning are affected by their decisions and transitions over time. This book, therefore, describes much more than an academic exercise. The findings are drawn from and have implications for the real world, with all its complexities and challenges. Consequently, the potential readership extends far beyond the academic community. It presents an important road map for providers, policymakers and individuals and their families who are facing these decisions either today or tomorrow.

I urge all readers to heed the observations and recommendations made by the authors in their concluding chapter. First, this book has raised as many questions as it has answered and provides a research agenda for others to pursue. Second, a dialogue between researchers, housing providers, policymakers and the general public must occur if we are to move beyond applied research to sound policy and practice.

Preface

We are on the brink of a national crisis: the absence of sufficient supportive housing arrangements for growing numbers of aging Americans. We
know little about the decision-making processes of individuals and couples as they face the specter or the reality of changing housing and health
care needs. Neither is there sufficient evidence about the implications for
health, well-being, and social integration of various housing choices, including aging in place. To address these issues, this monograph draws on data
from a panel survey of more than 800 older adults (ages 55 to 100) living
in a variety of housing arrangements in an upstate New York county—the
Pathways to Life Quality study. This study examines the factors associated
with life quality for respondents living on their own in the local community, as well as those in various housing arrangements (such as a continuing care retirement facility, an adult home, income-subsidized housing,
and senior apartments) and those making residential moves between 1997
and 1999 (the first two survey waves).

This book, like the *Pathways* study on which it is based, is a collaborative project of faculty and students at Cornell University and Ithaca
College. First conceived by John Krout and Phyllis Moen several years
ago, the book's chapters have evolved over time as the study has unfolded.
Recently, Elaine Wethington replaced Professor Moen as the book's coau-
thor. Thus, this volume reflects the focuses of individuals with differing
disciplinary backgrounds, substantive interests, and research approaches.
The longitudinal nature of the research has provided us with additional
insight into the relationship between housing decisions and quality of life.
This book focuses on how changes in health, well-being, and social integration, as well as satisfaction with housing and community are related to
the type of residential environment (or changes in that environment) in
which older people live. A second key focus is on the decision-making
process—the reasons for moving or staying in a residence as well as

factors that relate to planning and to successful transitions to new living environments. The authors have used the same data set, and that provides an important thread of continuity across chapters. Because the authors represent a wide variety of disciplines, the book offers an important multi-disciplinary vantage point from which to view the housing and life quality of older Americans.

Our research aims to improve understanding of the relationship between residential planning, type of residence and residential moves, and well-being among older adults. We also identify the implications of research findings concerning the planning for and timing of moves (or of aging in place) and their implications for life quality. It is impossible in a book of this length to discuss all of the findings of the *Pathways to Life Quality* study. We have pulled together findings central to understanding the relationship between housing or living environments and the quality of life. We have selected topics that should be particularly instructive for practitioners and consumers and that are applicable in other communities. These topics include how housing transitions and social, psychological, and health status affect each other; how aging in place unfolds in various housing situations; and how and why older adults come to change their living environment.

Each chapter follows a similar structure and includes the following sections: an introduction; a review of literature pertinent to its topic; a discussion of any methodological issues involved in its analysis; findings; implications of the findings for research, housing policy, consumers and practice; and a summary and conclusion. Authors focus on the correlates of living environment and residential change for a number of topics. The topics include: moving behavior and plans; the relationship of environmental features and place attachment; role identities; social relationships, participation, and integration; health and activity patterns; health and social service use; psychological well-being; and adjustment to life events. Each chapter also includes residential comparisons and looks at changes over time if the data are available. Chapters have been organized into six sections.

In the first section, Krout and Wethington introduce the rationale for the book and present an overview of the need to examine these topics. They lay out the context of the book with a review of previous research and theory on the impact of living environments on older adults, including the work of Lawton, Lawton and Nahemow, Golant, and others. This chapter also provides an overview of the goals and research design of the *Pathways to*

Life Quality study, including sampling, data collection, variables, measurement, and types of residential environments included in the study.

The second section includes two chapters. Chapter 2, by Krout, Holmes, Erickson, and Wolle, provides an overview of the literature that deals with residential relocation behavior and attitudes among older adults. It then presents data from the *Pathways* study concerning the reasons given for moving into a continuing care retirement community (CCRC) by its first cohort of residents. The reasons most likely to be identified include the on-site availability of care for self and spouse, regardless of level of disability; freedom from having to worry about and do home maintenance; and desire to avoid being a burden to adult children. They also report on variations in expectations of moving in the future, based on current residence as well as anticipated type of living arrangements. Aging in place, with or without major home adaptations, is the most likely future housing scenario, whereas living with family is given a very low probability. Chapter 3, by Eshelman, Evans, and Utamura, examines the relationship between the features of community housing and satisfaction with that housing. Their findings provide insights into the types of features that promote a feeling of home and that could be used by planners of senior residences. Specifically, they compare the impact of features that augment physical functioning for aging people, to those that allow residents to personalize their surroundings with objects that provide personal meaning.

Section 3 of the volume focuses on the changes in social roles, role identities, social participation, and social integration that aging people experience in various residential settings and in response to relocation. In chapter 4, Moen, Dempster-McClain, Erickson, and Boyce examine role participation and role identity over time, looking in particular at how specific role changes and relocation in general affect changes in role identities. Previous research on roles and role identities has tended to conflate the two concepts. The authors, however, demonstrate that role participation and role identity are separate concepts that need to be distinguished in research and in practice. In the subsequent chapter (chapter 5), Erickson and Moen consider changes in social integration over time, considering separately structural integration (the number of roles that people hold) and psychological integration (the perception of being involved in meaningful social activity). Their findings indicate that recent relocation and the particular residential setting are associated with changes in structural integration and psychological integration across time.

Section 4 turns to a consideration of health, health service utilization, and social service utilization. In chapter 6, Holmes, Beissner, Welsh, and Krout report that nonsenior housing residents are healthier than elders in senior housing and find considerable variation in reports of chronic health conditions and disability based on type of housing. Given the complexity of factors related to health, they find it difficult to determine the impact of the living environment itself on health and disability status. Holmes, Krout, and Wolle look at patterns of use of a variety of community-based services in chapter 7. They find relatively high levels of overall use, especially for residents of "service-rich" senior housing. However, use of individual services varies considerably ("senior center," "transportation," and "homemaker" are the most commonly used), and it changes for individuals over time.

Section 5 shifts to a consideration of psychological well-being and adjustment over time, and how they differ in the context of stressful life events, social and psychological resources, declines in health, and specific residential settings. In chapter 8, Wethington examines the distribution of stressful life events, chronic stressors, and onset of increasing health problems on the basis of residential setting, recent relocation, and three age groups (the young-old, middle-old, and oldest old). Theoretical perspectives on stressful life events predict that loss events should increase as people age. On the other hand, survival perspectives suggest that those who survive to a ripe old age may begin to experience fewer events, including onsets of illness. Wethington finds that the number of events experienced by the three age groups is relatively constant, but that there are differences in the experience of events, chronic difficulties, and onsets of illness according to residential setting. Residents of facilities that provide fewer services report significantly more chronic stressors other than those involving health. Residents of all senior housing facilities (including those providing a larger number of services) have experienced more recent health declines, which may have prompted their moves to those facilities. Residential settings, however, are associated with significant reductions in perceived health and personal mastery, adjusting for recent life stressors, preexisting health status, personal mastery, and levels of social integration. Changes in perceived health are also predicted by onsets of new illnesses and by declining personal mastery, both of which are more common among residents of senior facilities.

In chapter 9, Boyce, Wethington, and Moen turn to an examination of changes in psychological well-being across time, utilizing three different measures of well-being. Previous research into well-being in old age has come to conflicting conclusions about whether increasing age is associated with a diminished sense of well-being. In the so-called paradox of well-being, many older people maintain stable well-being in the face of increasing number of life events, declining health, and shrinking social networks and resources. The unique contribution of the chapter is its consideration of this topic in the context of residential settings and recent relocation. The authors find that residents of senior housing that offers fewer resources show the most negative profiles on all three measures of psychological well-being. However, they do not show significant decreases in well-being between the two waves, indicating that there are important preexisting differences in the well-being of those who move to different types of residential facilities that may help explain any differences in their overall adjustment to relocation. They also find that recent life events and the onset of new illnesses significantly reduce life satisfaction among older people, but do not have a long-lasting impact on levels of positive and negative affect, controlling for preexisting levels of psychological and social resources.

Finally, Section 6 looks in greater detail at all the chapters in terms of their implications for policy and practice and provides a final chapter that summarizes the book as a whole. In chapter 10, Krout and Pillemer identify and discuss a number of questions about the implications of the research. These questions include the quality-of-life indicators of particular importance for housing and long-term care policy and services; the implications of health and disability patterns of older adults living in congregate housing; the services that are needed and used by older adults living in various settings; the changes experienced by older adults when they relocate to congregate housing; and the information that would be useful to older adults in making housing-related decisions. The concluding chapter (chapter 11), by Wethington and Krout, identifies common themes that emerge throughout the book and raises research questions for the future.

One important common theme relates to how socioeconomic and other resources constrain strategies for coping with declining health and mobility as one ages, including relocating to facilities that may help offset health declines. Facilities that offer services to help offset the impact of declines in health and mobility are available only to older persons with significant financial resources. A second common theme relates to the ways in which the needs and desires of those who have relocated to senior facilities change over time. Those older people who plan ahead and relocate before health decline overtakes them may find that the facility no longer fits their needs as they become less interested in leisure amenities and more interested in access to long-term care. On the other hand, those who relocate to a senior facility after their health has declined may locate to a different type of facility. A third common theme is that changes in health and informal social support may lead to relocation. These changes are not necessarily mitigated by the potential social benefits of congregate housing or by services provided in those facilities if health has declined to the point where social participation has become difficult.

These themes in turn raise new questions about the future design of long-term care facilities. An increasing number of people who lack supportive family ties are approaching retirement. Smaller family sizes, increasing rates of divorce, and the prevalence of stepfamily living suggest that many baby boomers will enter old age with small or nonexistent family networks. Social and financial planners are busy marketing long-term care insurance, retirement plans, and other financial safeguards to the most financially advantaged baby boomers. Housing planners are already designing retirement communities that cater to upper-income elders. How will our society deal with aging people who cannot afford to relocate to facilities that offer services that assist in the activities of daily living? If there is indeed evidence that facilities can improve the functioning of older adults who need assistance and care in performing the activities of life, how do we make them available to those who cannot afford them?

Second, given that most older people plan to live at home as long as possible—and that some will never willingly relocate to congregate residential settings—how do we provide services for those who wish to remain in their homes? How do we provide incentives for people to plan ahead for long-term care needs?

The primary audience for this book is academic researchers, educators, graduate and perhaps advanced undergraduate students, and housing professionals, including developers, planners, and managers. A secondary audience is older consumers and their families and community planners who are interested in local housing options. The book is useful as a reference work on housing and older adults, particularly for scholars and practitioners interested in how to study the impact of housing environments on the quality of life of older persons. We believe it also has application as a primary or supplementary textbook for courses at the graduate or advanced undergraduate level; it would be appropriate for courses on housing and aging as well as those concerned with quality of life among older adults.

In conclusion, this book is a testament to the value of interinstitutional, multidisciplinary, and interdisciplinary collaborative research into aging. The blending of faculty, students, and staff of differing disciplinary backgrounds led us to ask and examine questions in exciting and creative ways. Variables not generally used in research on housing issues, such as life events, daily activities, and perceived role identities, are applied creatively here to understand the dynamic processes that lead to relocation in old age.

JAK
EW
Ithaca, New York

Acknowledgments

Many people have contributed to this book and helped move it from an idea to a reality. Our *Pathways to Life Quality* study advisory committee provided critical and crucial advice on the research design, especially on data collection and respondent recruitment. Committee members were Robert Butler, Thomas Grape, Vernon Greene, Sy Kingsly, Nancy Spears, Robyn Stone, and Roy Unger. Gordon Streib's observations and suggestions as a project evaluator were extremely helpful for our understanding of how to improve our research.

A large number of staff members were responsible for the day-to-day operation of the *Pathways* study and put together the data files on which the book is based. These staff members were Alice Boyce, Carrie Chalmers, Rachel Dickinson, Eileen Driscoll, Mary Ann Erickson, Heidi Holmes, Joanne Jordan, Aparajita Maitra, Jessie Moore, Jean Oggins, Alison Weinstein, Sue Welch, Carol Whitlow, and Sarah Wolle. Larry Clarkberg is also to be thanked for his excellent editorial contributions to this manuscript. In addition, approximately 120 Ithaca College and Cornell University students conducted the in-person interviews or coded data for the *Pathways* study.

We also would like to acknowledge Phyllis Moen for her important work as an initial coprincipal investigator on the *Pathways* study and coeditor of this book. And we would like to recognize the support given to the *Pathways* project by administrators at both of our institutions. At Cornell University, Francille Firebaugh and Patsy Brannon, the former and current deans of the College of Human Ecology, have supported the financial, material, and other program needs for *Pathways to Life Quality* and its home, the Bronfenbrenner Life Course Center. At Ithaca College, former Dean of the School of Health Sciences and Human Performance, Richard Miller and former President, James J. Whalen, provided unwavering support for gerontology program initiatives. In addition, this book would not have been possible without the support The Atlantic Philanthropies (USA) Inc. provided for the *Pathways to Life Quality* study.

Last, but not least, we would like to thank David and Bobbi for their forbearance in the face of all the inevitable interruptions that editing a book brings to home life.

SECTION 1

Introduction

CHAPTER 1

Introduction

John A. Krout and Elaine Wethington

Since 1997, researchers at Ithaca College and Cornell University have been collecting longitudinal data in an upstate New York county to examine the relationship between different types of housing environments and well-being among older adults. Called *Pathways to Life Quality*, the study also allows researchers to investigate the decision-making process involved in residential relocation, its outcomes, and how these change over time. An important goal of this book is to identify and discuss the implications of these researchers' findings for older adults, housing planners, and practitioners. This introductory chapter discusses the background and context of the book. It provides an overview of the need for research on the housing arrangements and transitions of older adults and offers a brief survey of the literature that deals with what we know about the relationship between housing and well-being. Next, we discuss the goals of the *Pathways to Life Quality* study and the major questions it sought to answer. We give a brief overview of the study's conceptual orientation and uniqueness as well as a summary of the research design, including sampling, data collection, measurement, and analysis.

CONTEXT AND SIGNIFICANCE OF THE BOOK

More Americans are living longer than ever before, with the number of the 85-and-over population expanding particularly rapidly (six times faster than the rest of the population). These demographic trends have been accompanied by a growing recognition that the residential preferences and requirements of individuals change with increasing age, in tandem with changes in their health, functional ability, and lifestyle choices.

The overwhelming preference of older adults is to stay in their homes as long as possible (Harper & Bayer, 2000). When disability makes independent living no longer possible, people have had to choose between living in their current home with assistance (aging in place) or moving to a nursing home. Nursing homes clearly are not the preferred living environment for individuals, regardless of age. Moreover, nursing homes place heavy economic burdens on families and, increasingly, on federal and state programs such as Medicare and Medicaid.

To bridge this lack of fit between the residential preferences and needs of older adults and current housing options, an increasing number of residential alternatives have become available. Along with skilled nursing homes for those with severe functional impairments, we find senior apartments that offer no or very few supportive services and others that have a more service-rich environment. Some older adults have moved to retirement communities in which residence and sometimes home ownership is restricted to people in their fifties or older. These communities usually consist of townhouses or single-family dwellings and often have centers that offer programs such as social and community events, classes, and exercise opportunities. Other types of housing include board-and-care homes, adult homes, and assisted-living facilities, formats that provide a range of supportive individual and congregate services, including personal care but generally not medical services. In addition, continuing care retirement communities (CCRCs) that provide a variety of residential options ranging from independent living to skilled nursing care in the same campus-like setting have become increasingly widespread.

Just as the demographic makeup of the individuals who choose each type of residential option differs, so the environments they live in are variously designed to provide social support and continuity in care as people age and experience functional declines. In the best of circumstances, these types of housing allow the individual as much independence as possible while providing services that are responsive to shifting health and social needs. The presumption is that this support allows for a better (or at least a different) quality of life as one ages in place than is found in other living situations.

However, little is known about the long-term experiences of older adults living in these various types of congregate settings, how individuals successfully make the transition to communal living, and how their experiences compare to those of older individuals residing in the community. Individuals choosing these newer types of residential environments are pathfinders exploring uncharted terrain. We know little about their goals and expectations for the future or about the forces and experiences that facilitate successful transition and a meaningful, high-quality life in a residential environment. Nor do we understand the long-term consequences of remaining in one's own residence—how does this choice affect an older individual's health, health care usage and costs, lifestyle, and social integration? We need information about these issues so older adults and their family members can be informed about the kinds of experiences various housing options are likely to provide and so housing professionals and policy makers can better plan for the housing needs and preferences of a growing and increasingly diverse older population.

This book, then, examines issues that will become even more pivotal as we enter the 21st century. When is the optimal time to make a residential move, both in terms of psychological adjustment and health? Which housing arrangement is most conducive to health, life quality, and reduced health care costs? What are the processes by which residential moves are decided upon or timed, or the cost and benefits of not moving? This book addresses these questions, questions that have become more pressing as the nation begins the 21st century.

PREVIOUS RESEARCH AND THEORY

As most people age they experience declines in their functional abilities (sensory, psychomotor, etc.) and become both more dependent on their environments and more susceptible to negative outcomes if these environments are inappropriate for them (Choi, 1996). By environment, we mean the range of living spaces, from bedrooms, bathrooms, and living rooms to types of housing and residences, such as single-family dwelling units, apartments, and assisted-living, including the common spaces found within and near dwelling units and in communities as a whole. As more people live longer and age in place in an increasingly diverse number of settings, the question of how well environments facilitate and support physical, psychological, and social well-being takes on greater significance for individuals, families, communities, and the framers of social policy. Another key issue is the degree to which a living environment functions to maintain an individual's independence, autonomy, and choice (Birren, Lubben, Rowe, & Deutchman, 1991).

For almost 50 years, gerontologists have recognized that their living environments have significant impact on the behavior and well-being of older adults (Lawton, Windley, & Byerts, 1982; Scheidt & Windley, 1998). These person-environment theories of aging have built on Lewin's (1951) observation that behavior is a function of the interaction between the person and the environment. The best-known application of this framework is the ecological model of aging, Lawton and Nahemow's (1973) classic competence-press model. This model postulates that the response an environmental press (or stimulus) elicits from an individual is determined by that person's level of competence (biological, sensorimotor, perceptual, and cognitive), and the outcome of the interaction between the two can be either behavioral or psychological. Lawton and Nahemow further argue that the effect of a given press increases as the individual's competence decreases (the environmental docility hypothesis). A person's well-being and behavior are a result of the balance or lack thereof between the two. This approach directs our attention to the consideration of both the nature of the environment and the competencies of the individual as well as to the behavioral and psychological outcomes.

This model has been reformulated in response to criticisms that the model was too environmentally deterministic (Lawton, 1989) and so as to allow recognition that environments include resources as well as demands (Scheidt & Windley, 1998). Other scholars have attempted to place greater emphasis on the individual as well. Golant (1991, 1998) has formulated a perspective that gives more attention to the individual, and that is relevant to our work. His whole-person perspective identifies 18 individual characteristics that affect adaptation to housing. These characteristics include many of the variables examined in the *Pathways* study: personality traits; social identity; preference for privacy; competence; and life satisfaction. And Rowles (1984, 1988) has developed an approach to explain the experience of being old in rural Appalachian communities.

Over the years, gerontologists have looked at a wide range of topics concerning the relationship between where an older person lives and his or her well-being. Most of this work has examined the experiences of older people in various types of housing, usually congregate. Topics include the impact of nursing homes and other types of housing (e.g., low-income, assisted living) (Birren, Lubben, Rowe, & Deutchman, 1991; Scheidt & Windley, 1998); the impact of age segregation in retirement communities (Altman, Lawton, & Wohlwill, 1984; Burby & Rohe, 1990); involuntary relocation of people into institutions; voluntary relocation, including Sunbelt migration (Longino & Fox, 1995; Scheidt & Windley, 1998; U.S. Department of Commerce, 1998); how older adults relate to, use, and perceive neighborhoods (Altman, Lawton, & Wohlwill, 1984; Porter et al., 1995); the impact of specific design features found in individual living or communal and public spaces (Byerts, Howell, & Pastalan, 1979); the aging experience in rural versus urban communities (Coward & Krout, 1998; Gesler, DeFriese, & Rabiner, 1998; Krout, 1986; Zimmer & Chapell, 1997); and the public- and private-sector roles in providing housing for older adults (Anikeeff & Mueller, 1998; Liebig, 1995).

In terms of residential transitions, many previous studies have reported negative outcomes of moves to congregate settings, but some have reported on the positive benefits such moves can bring (Golant, 1998). Recently, researchers have acknowledged that most older adults do not relocate, even as their health and their economic and social situations change. Thus, an increasing number of studies have looked at topics such as aging in place; naturally occurring retirement communities (NORCs) that can result when younger persons move out of an area; and the use of home modification and in-home services to maximize independence and put off relocation (Golant, 1998).

Our interest, however, lies not in further specifying particular theories about aging and the environment, but rather in using existing theories to examine larger questions: the role housing plays in the behavior and well-being (physical, psychological, and social) of older adults; the causes and consequences of housing transitions; and the role housing plays in maintaining well-being over time, particularly as older people experience life-course transitions. The reasons for and outcomes of relocation by older adults to congregate settings have received some attention from gerontologists. Less attention has been given to examining the causes of variations in how successfully older individuals age over time in differing housing arrangements.

In sum, our review of the literature indicates that a small number of researchers have examined the relationship between the environment and aging. However, relatively little information is available about residential differences for older adults, including the reasons they change residences, and about how such residential transitions impact well-being. We know little about the circumstances under which relocation promotes more successful aging in place. The research that has been done consists almost entirely of cross-sectional studies, so almost nothing is known of how housing environments relate to changes in the attitudes, behaviors, and needs of older adults over time. The work to date has been largely unidisciplinary and has not applied the perspectives of multiple disciplines. Finally, researchers have rarely attempted to draw out the implications of their findings for aging individuals, facility planners, and social policy makers. Researchers need to provide consumers and housing professionals with information about the consequences of relocation and the changes over time that can be expected to unfold in various settings.

THE CCRC PILOT PROJECT

Between 1995 and 1997, the Gerontology Institute at Ithaca College and the Bronfenbrenner Life Course Center at Cornell University collaborated on a project that served as the first phase of the research reported in this book. Working with limited funds but a great deal of enthusiasm from faculty and students on both campuses, this project was designed to provide preliminary data about the changes experienced by individuals in a CCRC and to identify the factors related to successful transitions to this type of residence.

This pilot study included 101 individuals who were among the initial group of older adults who had made the commitment to move into a new CCRC being built in an upstate community. The director of the facility contacted all 204 individuals who had signed contracts by June 1995 and asked them to return a postcard to the researchers if they were willing to participate in the study. This was a baseline, pre-move study designed to explore a wide variety of issues, including the decision to move, current housing quality, lifestyle, nutrition, and health. The data were collected through the use of both self-administered surveys and interviews. Detailed research instruments were developed to collect a large array of data: demographics; health and nutrition; characteristics of previous residences; exercise and activity; work history; availability of and contact with social networks; community involvement; perceived life quality; and a number of measures of psychological well-being. Much of the initial analysis looked at the reasons for relocation to the CCRC; psychological and social relationships; health and activities, and the use of those services; and the characteristics of current housing and respondents' assessment of it. These data were to be used as baseline information in examination of the changes that occurred over time.

Several aspects of this study make it unique. First, it is a research partnership between Ithaca College (a primarily undergraduate, comprehensive college) and Cornell University (a large PhD-granting research university). Second, student involvement was a key element of the project. Approximately 125 undergraduate and graduate students participated in the project, either conducting interviews or working on data analysis.

Third, the pilot project brought together a dozen research and teaching faculty members from a variety of disciplinary backgrounds, including sociology, psychology, marketing, design and environmental analysis, and family and human development. Through this initial pilot research we discovered the value of cross-disciplinary, collaborative research and the synergy and enduring commitment of our research team.

Convinced of the potential of this collaboration, Professors Krout and Moen applied for and secured funding for five years to continue the study of the CCRC residents and to include residents of other congregate facilities (excluding nursing homes) as well older adults living in a range of settings in the community. This 5-year time frame was considered to be phase one of a 10- to 20-year panel study, as tracking older individuals' housing patterns and modes of adaptation over the course of life clearly calls for a longitudinal design, including several cohorts of individuals confronting housing choices and transitions. This project was called the *Pathways to Life Quality* study.

THE *PATHWAYS TO LIFE QUALITY* STUDY

The *Pathways to Life Quality* study has three main goals:

- To investigate the effects of various residential settings on the health, well-being, and life quality of a sample of older Americans in an upstate New York community;
- To assess the decision-making choices regarding residential moves of older Americans, including their timing, degree of choice, and the factors influencing residential changes or stability; and
- To increase the knowledge about gerontology and the research skills of several cohorts of faculty and students and provide them with opportunities to interact with older adults.

This book focuses on the first two goals. Thus, the impact on students, faculty, and curriculum and teaching is not discussed. However, it is noteworthy that approximately 125 students and two dozen faculty members participated in the data collection, analysis, and dissemination of findings. The *Pathways* study has become a focal point for multidisciplinary research into aging on both campuses.

As noted earlier, the *Pathways* study expanded the pilot project by studying older adults living in a wider variety of settings over a longer period of time. The housing facilities included a number of small, rural senior-apartment complexes; an adult home that relocated to a new facility that included apartments for independent living; a high-rise apartment complex built in accordance with Section 8 of the U.S. Department fo Housing and Urban Development (HUD); and an apartment house for low- to middle-income seniors. Also, additional faculty members became involved in the research. The disciplines represented in this book include gerontology, sociology, psychology, human development, physical therapy, architecture, and design and environmental analysis.

FACILITY DESCRIPTIONS

In order to expand the usefulness of the research, we broadened the variety of living environments examined as much as possible so as to include congregate living facilities in both the urban and the rural parts of the study area. Each type of facility is described briefly.

CONTINUING CARE RETIREMENT COMMUNITY

The CCRC in this study is a not-for-profit life care retirement community designed for people 65 or older who are in good physical and mental health. The CCRC, by virtue of its fees, which include an entrance fee and monthly apartment or cottage costs, is affordable only to a limited segment of the population. Located in a rural college community, it has attracted primarily professionals, including many who had worked at the town's academic

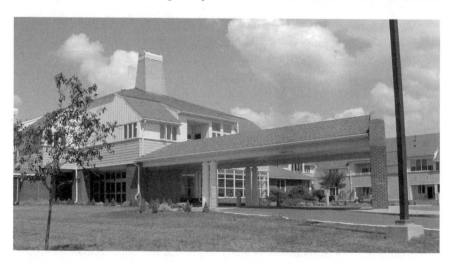

Figure 1.1 Continuing care retirement community.

institutions. The CCRC offers a choice of apartment and cottage sizes, including studios and one- and two-bedroom spaces. In addition to providing meals, housekeeping, linen services, maintenance, groundskeeping, a library, and space for exercise and recreation (including a pool), it offers an on-site health center that provides short- and long-term care. Care includes 24-hr-a-day skilled nursing, assisted living, the services of a doctor, rehabilitation therapy, a social services staff, a pharmacy, and home care.

INDEPENDENT AND ASSISTED LIVING FACILITY

Until 1998, this facility was an 80-resident adultcare home in which most residents received assisted-living services such as personal care and meals. In November 1998, the adult home relocated to a new facility that also included 100 independent-living apartments—a mix of studio and one- and two-bedroom units. The residents of the independent-living section can receive services such as two meals a day, linen and housekeeping, groundskeeping, a library, a chapel, an exercise room, a pool, a greenhouse, and craft rooms. This residential facility was designed to incorporate an intergenerational partnership with a college nearby. Students and faculty from the college are involved in internships, recreational activities, research projects, volunteer work, and a variety of intergenerational programs. A social worker is on the staff, as is a part-time chaplain.

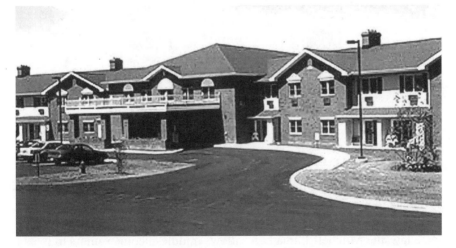

Figure 1.2 Independent and Assisted Living Facility

SECTION 8 APARTMENT COMPLEX

This two-building high-rise with approximately 235 residents is part of a rent-subsidized, Section 8 HUD program for low-income individuals and has been in the community for 30 years. For most of its existence, it was for seniors only, but recent changes in federal laws and regulations have allowed the residency of other low-income populations, including individuals with mental illness or chemical-addiction problems. Meals are not provided, although many residents take part in the local home-delivered meals program. There is a staff on site, including the housing manager, a social worker, and a maintenance crew. There is also a very active tenant council. The building is conveniently located on the city bus route and is within walking distance of a city park and a shopping plaza.

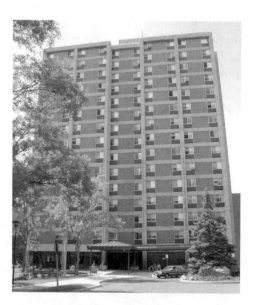

Figure 1.3 A section 8 apartment complex.

LOW- AND MIDDLE-INCOME APARTMENT COMPLEX

This facility is open to low- and middle-income seniors older than 62 and is managed by a nonprofit organization. HUD provides a low interest rate on the mortgage of the building, which was built in 1971. A New York state law, the Mitchell-Lama Law, allows middle-income seniors to live in the facility and pay rent equal to 30% of their incomes. Located in a small

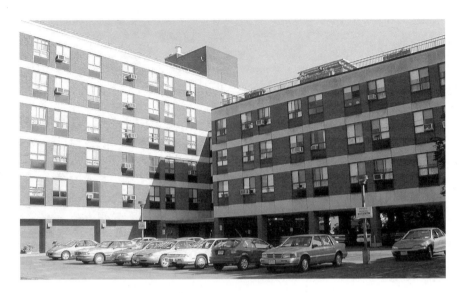

Figure 1.4 A low-and middle-income apartment complex.

urban community, this facility has studio and one-bedroom apartments with 9 staff members and 111 residents. The parent organization helps to support the residence by providing evening meals at reduced cost to the residents. There are a facility manager, a groundskeeper and maintenance worker, and two administrative assistants on staff. The building also features a rooftop garden and promenade deck and a recreation room.

RURAL SENIOR HOUSING

Seven small rural facilities dedicated to housing senior residents are included in the study. The majority of these facilities are managed by local housing authorities and certified through the U.S. Federal Public Housing regulations. The facility managers are part-time employees and may supervise three separate facilities. There are no on-site health or support services, but residents do benefit from small-town life in that the local grocery stores will make home deliveries and the local home-health nurses have keys to the buildings. Many of these facilities have chairlifts but no elevators. All have some sort of community recreation room, and emergency call buttons are found in each apartment.

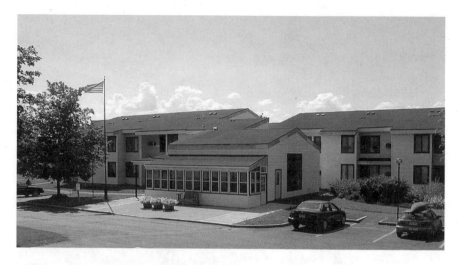

Figure 1.5 A rural senior housing.

NON-FACILITY GROUPS

In addition to the groups of individuals living in congregate facilities, two groups of older adults living in the community are included in the study. The first includes approximately 100 older individuals not living in a facility but on the waiting list of the independent/assisted-living facility. This group gives researchers the opportunity to follow older adults before and after their move to a congregate facility, as was the case with the CCRC sample. The second is a random sample of approximately 400 county residents (60 and older) not living in facilities.

The wide range of living environments in the study provides a basis for comparing and contrasting experiences. It also allows for comparison of various kinds of living environments. The community sample is key to understanding how individuals moving into a residential community may differ from their neighbors who choose not to do so. This sample includes great variability in housing characteristics that could influence health and well-being and also permits assessment of the relative advantages of aging in place as compared to the alternatives that have recently emerged. In addition, the sample allows the exploration of the impact of age, as it includes people as young as 60, whereas other residential options restrict entry until 62 or 65, and the majority of current residents are in their mid-70s or older. Because of the expense of some of the residential alternatives we examined, this community sample also increased the range of income levels studied, thus allowing exploration of this important factor. It also allowed us to collect data on individuals *before* they made any residential changes and to follow them through their decision-making process. The significance and power of the analysis of many of the issues examined, such as stress over time, are greater because of the number of individuals in the community sample.

SAMPLE

We made a priori decisions at the time of planning the research to exclude from the study individuals in nursing homes and those with dementia or levels of confusion that would prevent completion of the interview. Also, it was not possible to interview individuals who were completely deaf. In the initial recruitment phone call, an attempt was made to screen for these conditions. Screening for cognitive competency was also done by means of an examination of the responses to the first questions in the actual interview—the day and date, the type of residence, and the name of town of residence. During the initial recruitment call, interviewers also made sure the person met the basic study criteria of being 60 years old or older and a resident of the county being studied. The decision to study residents from only one county was based partly on practicality, but also on the desire to include students and faculty in as many phases of the research as possible. Because the research design called for personal interviews and home observations to be conducted every 2 years, the cost of going outside the county was considered prohibitive. Limitations on the generalizability of the research findings are outweighed by the detailed longitudinal data we have been able to collect.

In most of the facilities, we were unable to obtain a list of all residents due to confidentiality concerns, so we were not able to determine how representative the achieved samples were. With the cooperation of facility administrators, we tried to recruit all potential participants by means of flyers, presentations by faculty and staff, sing-alongs, and ice cream socials. The random community sample consisted of 3,000 names (well in excess of the number needed) drawn randomly from a pool of 13,197 names compiled from three sources: purchased age-targeted lists of county residents from Survey Sampling, Inc.; county voter registration records; and the mailing lists of county senior citizens' organizations. This pool included very nearly the entire population of those 60 years and older in the target county. Potential participants were contacted first by a mailing that included a letter from the principal investigators and a brochure explaining the study. Phone calls were then made sequentially, starting with the first randomly selected name. Recruitment of participants was carried out by telephone. Given the recruitment of an individual, we then made every effort to recruit the spouse or partner of that individual too, whenever such a partner was present. Decisions regarding the inclusion or exclusion of spouses and partners in analyses and methods to ensure that models take into account the nonindependence of individuals within families are noted in each analysis.

There is an excellent correspondence between the demographic composition of the *Pathways* randomly drawn community sample and the target county population aged 60 and older in the 1990 census. An examination of age distribution, race, sex, marital status, and income in the random sample and the census confirms the representative nature of the study sample. For details on this comparison and other aspects of the *Pathways* research and sampling design, see Henderson and Oggins (1999).

In addition, as a result of news coverage of the *Pathways* project prior to recruitment, 41 individuals in the target county general community volunteered to participate in the study. Because these participants were not randomized, we regard them as a separate sample, and they are distinguished from the random sample by a code in the data files. Decisions regarding the inclusion of this sample in analyses and the need to distinguish it from the random sample are also noted in each analysis.

In wave 1 (interviewed in 1997), two thirds of the individuals in the total sample are female, and slightly more than half (56%) of them are married. The average age is 74 and the average number of limitations reported is 1.7. Three quarters of them report some or a full college education, and one third note graduate school or a graduate degree. Concomitantly, incomes are relatively high, with one half of the sample reporting annual household incomes of $40,000 or more. Two years later, at the time of wave 2 (Table 1.2), the average age (not surprisingly) is slightly over 76 and the average number of limitations increases to 2. The percentage of female declines slightly and the percentage of those married drops to just over half. Education and income levels remain basically the same.

The characteristics of the older adults in the study varied considerably bassed on their housing. Table 1.1 and 1.2 present the sample characteristics of respondents who participated in both waves of interviews at both Wave 1 and Wave 2, based on Wave 2 housing arrrangement. For example, in wave 1, the percentage of females ranges from a low of 61% among

TABLE 1.1 Sample Characteristics at Wave 1 by Housing Type

	Community[a]	Service-poor		Service-rich	Movers
		Rural	City		
	(*n* = 384)	(*n* = 58)	(*n* = 78)	(*n* = 127)	(*n* = 39)
Age	72	78	77	77	81
	(±7.5)	(±6.8)	(±8.6)	(±6.4)	(±6.1)
Gender					
Men	39%	14%	17%	36%	28%
Women	61%	83%	83%	64%	72%
Marital status					
Unmarried	34%	86%	86%	37%	62%
Married	66%	14%	14%	63%	38%
Income					
< $20,000	20.4%	87.3%	79.6%	2.5%	15.2%
$20,000–39,999	27.1%	12.7%	18.5%	5.1%	54.5%
$40,000–74,999	32.2%	0.0%	1.9%	44.9%	30.3%
$75,000 and up	20.4%	0.0%	0.0%	47.5%	0.0%
Education					
High school or less	23.8%	54.4%	52.6%	2.4%	25.6%
College	40.9%	42.1%	36.8%	40.5%	48.7%
Graduate degree	35.4%	3.5%	10.5%	57.1%	25.6%
Self-rated health	7.8	6.4	6.6	7.4	6.9
	(±1.8)	(±2.2)	(±2.3)	(±2.0)	(±1.8)
Activity limitations	1.0	3.4	2.6	1.4	3.0
	(±1.2)	(±3.5)	(±2.8)	(±2.5)	(±3.1)
Number of children	3.1	3.3	2.9	2.9	2.0
	(±1.7)	(±3.3)	(±1.8)	(±2.1)	(±1.2)

[a]   Includes randomly selected individuals and spouses, but not community volunteers.

community residents to a high of 83% among service-poor facility residents and 100% among assisted-living residents. The percentage of individuals with graduate degrees ranges from a high of 57% in the CCRC to zero in the HUD apartments. Considerable variation is found for the other characteristics as well. Consequently, we pay particular attention in our analyses to how these measures interact with measures of life change and life quality.

Congregate housing respondents living in the CCRC are included in the service-rich category because of the robustness of on-site services and

TABLE 1.2 Sample Characteristics at Wave 2 by Housing Type

| | Community[a] | Service-poor | | Service-rich | Movers |
| | | Rural | City | | |
	(n = 384)	(n = 58)	(n = 78)	(n = 127)	(n = 40)
Age	74	80	80	80	83
	(±7.5)	(±6.8)	(±8.6)	(±6.3)	(±6.0)
Gender					
Men	39%	11%	17%	36%	26%
Women	61%	89%	83%	64%	74%
Marital Status					
Unmarried	34%	90%	91%	43%	62%
Married	66%	10%	9%	57%	38%
Income					
< $20,000	19.3%	85.7%	77.4%	0.0%	19.0%
$20,000–39,999	28.7%	14.3%	17.7%	13.9%	47.6%
$40,000–74,999	28.7%	0.0%	3.2%	29.7%	33.3%
$75,000 and up	23.2%	0.0%	1.6%	56.4%	0.0%
Education					
High school or less	24.0%	55.2%	47.4%	3.2%	25.6%
College	42.1%	41.4%	39.5%	42.2%	48.7%
Graduate degree	33.9%	3.4%	13.2%	54.5%	25.6%
Self-rated health	7.7	7	6.4	7.3	7.2
	(±2.0)	(±2.1)	(±2.4)	(±2.1)	(±1.7)
Activity limitations	1.4	3.4	3.3	2.2	3.5
	(±2.2)	(±3.3)	(±2.9)	(±2.9)	(±3.5)
Number of children	3.0	3.3	2.9	3.1	2.5
	(±1.7)	(±3.3)	(±1.8)	(±2.3)	(±1.3)

[a] Includes randomly selected individuals and spouses, but not community volunteers.

facilities. Those living in rural or urban subsidized housing are categorized as service-poor. In looking at the profiles of residents living in the various housing arrangements, differences can be seen in a number of areas. Those who live in service-poor housing, whether it is rural or within the city limits, have significantly lower levels of education and income, rate their health as poorer, and typically are not married. Those who moved during the period between the interviews are older than the other groups and rate their health as being poorer than do the service-rich facility residents and the community sample. Higher percentages of the community sample and the service-rich facility residents are married.

DATA COLLECTION

The research design for the study involves interviewing respondents every 2 years, with ongoing recruitment at the facilities and "refreshing" the community sample every other interviewing cycle. During 1997 and 1998 (wave 1), we interviewed 868 older adults. The group included 154 in the CCRC (95 of whom had been interviewed in 1995); 75 in the urban apartment complexes; 71 in the rural apartment complexes; 111 in the independent/assisted-living facility (101 on the independent-living waiting list and 10 in the adult home); and 457 in the community (including 416 who were randomly selected and 41 volunteers). During 1999 and 2000 (wave 2), we interviewed 790 older adults, including 727 interviewed in Wave 1. This group included 139 in the CCRC; 76 in the urban apartment complexes; 60 in the rural apartment complexes; 48 in the independent/assisted-living facility, and 3 in a new assisted-living facility; 59 in the independent-living waiting list; and 405 in the community (including 47 volunteers). The majority of our sample (92%) did not relocate between wave 1 and wave 2, but 8% of the sample did move, 40 to a senior-housing facility and 19 to locations within the community. We observed that 29% of those on the waiting list for the independent-living facility had moved there.

Of the 141 respondents not reinterviewed in wave 2, death had claimed 43 (31%), and 98 (69%) had withdrawn, were unreachable, or were unable to complete the wave 2 interview. A significant number of those who had withdrawn had done so because of poor health, not because of a lack of interest in the study. The retention rate between waves 1 and 2 was 85%, an excellent rate for a longitudinal study of this nature. We attribute this high rate to the outstanding efforts made by our staff and students to contact previous respondents. These efforts included maintaining contact with respondents by means of birthday and holiday cards. In addition, we examined all obituaries and death notices in the local paper to track mortality in the sample. We also searched for names of respondents who had moved out of the area in the Social Security Death Index. Respondents who had left the area were tracked and sent surveys for self-administration or were interviewed by phone. We note that the data from respondents who had died or did not continue in the study are still useful in some analyses. The majority of interviews (63%) were conducted by students from Ithaca College or Cornell University. Independent contractors and the *Pathways to Life Quality* staff conducted the remainder of the interviews.

MEASURES

The *Pathways to Life Quality* study collects information about a wide variety of characteristics and attributes of the individuals and their living environments.

A considerable number of standard scales have been integrated into the research instrument. Embedded in the interview are several published scales. Faculty and staff use these measures to track adjustment, psychological well-being, and respondents' views of their lives and levels of satisfaction. Included are the following scales:

* Lawton Attitude toward Aging (Lawton, 1975)
* MacArthur Control (Haidt & Rodin, 1995)
* Rosenberg Self-Esteem (Rosenberg, 1965)
* Pearlin Mastery (Pearlin & Schooler, 1978)
* Perceived Constraints (Lachman & Weaver, 1998)
* Purpose in Life (Ryff & Keyes, 1995)
* Social Provisions (Cutrona & Russell, 1987; Cutrona, Russell, & Rose, 1986)
* Positive and Negative Affect (Mroczek & Kolarz, 1998)
* Generativity (Rossi, 2001)

Also included are a series of questions about moving plans, housing, health and disability, exercise and activities, service use, social integration and role participation, and recent life events. The interviews thoroughly assess reasons for moving, as well as expectations of and plans for moving in the future. There are numerous questions about aspects of housing, including overall quality and satisfaction, as well as physical and psychological aspects of housing, such as space, personalization, design, health and safety features, and privacy. The health or disability of respondents (and their spouses, if applicable) are assessed using measures of perceived health and energy, recent onsets of physical illness, utilization of health services, sensory declines, and limitations in performing the activities of daily living. There are numerous measures of common social and physical activities, including exercise. We assessed awareness and use of services available for older people in the county. Social and role participation are represented by measures of frequency of interaction with neighbors, friends, families, and groups, including volunteer groups, as well as the degree to which participants rates these contacts as being important to their identities. We also ask respondents about recent social transitions, losses and other recent life events that may have caused stress.

In sum, this book contributes to understanding the long-term experiences of older adults living in various types of residential settings. Another goal of this project has been to apply a multidisciplinary approach to the process of relocation among older people. As a caution, we must acknowledge at the outset that the experiences of those in *Pathways to Life Quality* study may not generalize to all regions of the country, or to future generations of older people facing the same decisions.

Nevertheless, much can be learned from this study. Perhaps most important is the message that relocation is a complex decision, for the most part undertaken over a period of years rather than in a few months. Plans for relocation vary over the course of aging, with the younger-old trying to maximize a set of factors different from those faced by individuals whose health is declining. Psychological factors such as attachment to place, the identity and meaning invested in a personal residence, strong preferences for privacy, and the American expectation of self-reliance, even at the end of life, are relevant factors in making a decision to relocate. They are also relevant in understanding how to improve the quality of life in senior-housing facilities.

REFERENCES

Altman, I., Lawton, M. P., & Wohlwill, J. F. (Eds.). (1984). *Elderly people and the environment*. New York: Plenum.

Anikeeff, M. A., & Mueller, G. R. (Eds.). (1998). *Seniors housing*. Boston: Kluwer Academic.

Birren, J. E., Lubben, J. E., Rowe, J. C., & Deutchman, D. E. (Eds.). (1991). *Improving residential environments for frail elderly: Bridging the gap between theory and application*. San Diego, CA: Academic.

Burby, R. J., & Rohe, W. M. (1990). Providing for the housing needs of the elderly. *Journal of the American Planning Association*, 56(3), 324–338.

Byerts, T. O., Howell, S. C., & Pastalan, L. A. (Eds.). (1979). *Environmental context of aging: Life-style, environmental quality, and living arrangements*. New York: Garland STPM.

Choi, N. G. (1996). Older persons who move: Reasons and health consequences. *Journal of Applied Gerontology, 15*(3), 325–344.

Coward, R., & Krout, J. (1998). *Aging in rural settings*. New York: Springer.

Cutrona, C. E., Russell, D. W., & Rose, J. (1986). Social support and adaptation to stress by the elderly. *Journal of Psychology and Aging, 1*(1), 47–54.

Cutrona, C. E., & Russell, D. W. (1987). The provisions of social relationships and adaptation to stress. *Advances in Personal Relationships, 1,* 37–67.

Gesler, W. M., DeFriese, G. H., & Rabiner, D. J. (1998). *Rural health and aging research: Theory, methods, and practical applications.* Amityville, NY: Baywood.

Golant, S. M. (1991). Congregate housing for the elderly: Theoretical, policy, and programmatic responses. *Journal of Housing for the Elderly, 9*(1–2), 21–38.

Golant, S. M. (1998). Changing an older person's shelter and care setting: A model to explain personal and environmental outcomes. In R. J. Scheidt and P. G. Windley (Eds.), *Environment and aging: A focus on housing* (pp. 33–60). Westport, CT: Greenwood.

Haidt, J., & Rodin, J. (1995). Control and efficacy: An integrative review. In (Eds.), *A report to the John D. and Catherine T. MacArthur Foundation Program on Mental Health and Human Development* (pp. 1–79).

Harper, L., & Bayer, A-H. (2000). *Fixing to stay: A national survey on housing and home modification issues.* Washington, DC: AARP.

Henderson, C., & Oggins, J. (1999). *Pathways research and sampling design* (working paper number 7). Ithaca, NY: *Pathways to Life Quality Study.*

Krout, J. (1986). *The aged in rural America.* Westport, CT: Greenwoood.

Lachman, M. E., & Weaver, S. L. (1998). Sociodemographic variations in the sense of control by domain: Findings from the MacArthur studies of midlife. *Psychology and Aging, 13*(4), 553–562.

Lawton, M. P. (1975). The Philadelphia geriatric center morale scale: A revision. *Journal of Gerontology, 30*(1), 85–89.

Lawton, M. P., & Nahemow, L. (1973). Ecology and the aging process. In C. Eisdorfer and M. P. Lawton (Eds.), *Psychology of adult development and aging* (pp. 619–674). Washington, DC: American Psychological Association.

Lawton, M. P., Windley, P. G., & Byerts, T. O. (1982). *Aging and the environment: Theoretical approaches.* New York: Springer.

Lawton, M. P. (1989). Environmental proactivity and affect in older people. In S. Spacapan and S. Oskamp (Eds.), *Social psychology of aging* (pp. 135–164). Newbury Park, CA: Sage.

Lewin, K. (1951). *Field theory in social sciences.* New York: Harper & Row.

Liebig, P. S. (1995). State units on aging and housing for the elderly: Current roles and future implications. In L. A. Pastalan (Ed.), *Housing decisions for the elderly: To move or not to move* (pp. 67–84). New York: Haworth.

Longino, C. F., Jr., & Fox, R. A. (Eds.). (1995). *Retirement migration in America.* Houston, TX: Vacation.

Mroczek, D. K., & Kolarz, C. M. (1998). The effect of age on positive and negative affect: A developmental perspective on happiness. *Journal of Personality and Social Psychology, 75*(5), 1333–1349.

Pearlin, L. I., & Schooler, C. (1978). The structure of coping. *Journal of Health and Social Behavior, 19*(1), 2–21.

Porter, D. R., Brecht, S. B., Cory, L. E., Faigin, R. A., Gamzon, M., & Taber, S. L. (1995). *Housing for seniors: Developing successful projects.* Washington, DC: Urban Land Institute.

Rosenberg, M. (1965). *Society and the adolescent self-image.* Princeton, NJ: Princeton University.

Rossi, A. S. (2001). *Caring and doing for others.* Chicago: University of Chicago.

Rowles, G. D. (1984). Aging in rural environments. In I. Altman, M. P. Lawton, & J. F. Wohlwill (Eds.), *Elderly people and the environment* (pp. 129–157). New York: Plenum.

Rowles, G. D. (1988). What's rural about rural aging: An Appalachian perspective. *Journal of Rural Studies, 4*(2), 115–124.

Ryff, C. D., & Keyes, C. L. M. (1995). The structure of psychological well-being revisited. *Journal of Personality and Social Psychology, 69*(4), 719–727.

Scheidt, R. J., & Windley, P. G. (Eds). (1998). *Environment and aging theory: A focus on housing.* Westport, CT: Greenwood.

U.S. Department of Commerce. (1998). *Seasonality of moves and duration of residence* (Series P70, No. 66). Washington, DC: U.S.G.P.O.

Zimmer, A., & Chapell, N. (1997). Rural-urban differences in seniors' neighborhood preferences. *Journal of Housing for the Elderly, 12*(1–2), 105–124.

SECTION 2

Housing Decision Making, Satisfaction, and Adaptation

CHAPTER 2

Residential Relocation

John A. Krout, Heidi Holmes,
Mary Ann Erickson, and Sarah Wolle

R esearch clearly indicates that older adults prefer to remain in their current housing situation and that they are less likely to move than younger adults. Nonetheless, gerontologists have been interested in who among the elderly move, where they move, why they move, and what the consequences of their moving are for themselves and others. Some studies have looked at involuntary relocation to nursing homes (Thomasma, Yeaworth, & McCabe, 1990; Thorson, 1988), while others have focused on voluntary moves, especially migration after retirement (Longino & Fox, 1995). Retirement to the Sunbelt has also attracted some interest from gerontologists and others (Longino & Fox, 1995; U.S. Department of Commerce, 1998). Typically, researchers have reported data concerning the characteristics of movers versus nonmovers and their reasons for moving (Choi, 1996; Sommers & Rowell, 1992). Much less information has been collected about the impact of relocation on individuals using pre- and post-move longitudinal data, the changes over time experienced by movers versus nonmovers, and how these impacts and changes vary depending on the type of residential environment an older person moves to and from (Mutchler & Burr, 1991). In addition, few data exist on the expectations of older adults who move and the relative attraction various types of residential options hold for them.

As greater numbers of adults reach old age with additional financial resources, in better health, and with more education, and as the scope of housing options widens, we can expect more residential relocation among this population. Some recent data suggest that older adults have become increasingly mobile (Clark & Davies, 1990; Flynn, Longino, Wiseman, &

Biggar, 1985). However, little research is available to help planners, developers, and housing practitioners predict where and why existing and future cohorts of older people will want to move or the demand for various housing options when they do move (Pynoos & Liebig, 1995). Furthermore, the degree to which new housing alternatives may influence established moving patterns is unclear.

This chapter addresses these important topics with findings from the *Pathways to Life Quality* study. First, the chapter provides a brief overview of existing research into residential relocation among older adults. We focus in particular on what previous research has found about who moves to continuing care retirement communities (CCRCs) and other congregate settings, why they move, the quality-of-life changes that appear to be associated with moving, and how movers differ from nonmovers. We also report on what is known about older people's expectations of moving. Next, this chapter presents and discusses analyses of the actual and anticipated moving behavior of older adults in the *Pathways* study. The longitudinal nature of our study provides prospective data for some of the sample. That is, people are asked about moving plans or reasons for moving before, not after, they move. Finally, we discuss the implications of our findings for research, for housing policy and practice, and for older adults.

LITERATURE REVIEW

MOVING BEHAVIOR OF OLDER ADULTS

Several recent surveys have found that the vast majority of American adults do not want to move (AARP, 1996; Harper & Bayer, 2000). Older adults are more likely to be homeowners, who are less likely to move than renters (Longino, Jackson, Zimmerman, & Bradsher, 1991; Miller, Longino, Anderson, James, & Worley, 1999). They have also lived in their residences for many years and report high levels of attachment to their homes (U.S. Bureau of the Census, 1996). Most older adults move locally when they do relocate (U.S. Bureau of the Census, 1996). Census data indicate that approximately 1% of adults 65 and older moved to a different state, and 4 to 6% moved within their state between 1992 and 1993 (U.S. Bureau of the Census, 1996).

Migration patterns of older adults are not random. Previous researchers have detailed migration streams in which migrants from certain areas of the country often move to specific destinations and tend to go to places similar in size to the ones they've left (U.S. Bureau of the Census, 1996).

Migration to the Sunbelt by "snowbirds" leaving the Northeast and Midwest for states in the Southeast, West, or Southwest has received considerable attention in the past (Longino, 1990; Rogers, 1988). Traditional models of migration such as Lee's (1966) point to push-pull factors as causes of this migration. Push factors for older adults are generally not job related but may reflect decreases in financial resources due to retirement. The declining health of self or spouse and significant life events such as the loss of a spouse also operate as push factors (Choi, 1996; Colsher & Wallace, 1990; Pynoos & Golant, 1996). For example, Choi found that 60% of movers cited their own poor health or their spouse's poor health or death, whereas 25% cited money problems as reasons for moving. Pull factors often include being closer to family, as well as amenities such as nicer weather, better recreational opportunities, availability of health care, and lower costs of living (Hass & Serow, 1993; Loomis, Sorce, & Tyler, 1989). Choi found clear patterns of intrastate and interstate moving that are consistent with and expand upon Lee's model. Of those who moved to another state, 41.5% cited being close to family or friends and 10% cited amenities as the primary reasons for moving (pull factors). Participants who cited financial hardship (a push factor) as the primary reason for moving generally stayed within their home state.

However, not all previous research fits with the push-pull model. Sommers and Rowell (1992) report that health status was not associated with moving whereas Pastalan (1995) reports that older adults who move are generally healthier, wealthier, and better educated. Colsher and Wallace (1990) found that relocation was associated with poorer physical functional status, poorer self-perceived health status and life satisfaction, higher levels of depressive symptomatology and anxiety, death of a spouse, marriage of offspring, and having someone move in. These apparent inconsistencies suggest a complex picture of which older persons move and why. For example, poor health is associated with some moves but not others. As Litwak and Longino (1987) point out in their stage theory, migration among older adults may begin with moves to take advantage of amenities when health and economic resources are adequate, but evolve to moves toward family resources and eventually to formal long-term care options.

In addition to the causes of older migration and the characteristics of older movers, researchers have also occasionally looked at the consequences of residential relocation (Ferraro, 1983; Scheidt & Windley, 1998). There is a considerable amount of information about the consequences of moving to nursing homes but very little about the implications of relocating to other living arrangements. The paucity of literature that does exist indicates that moving late in life has a small but significant negative effect on health (Choi, 1996). Furthermore, those who are forced to move to congregate housing experience more unhappiness, dissatisfaction, anxiety, and declines in health than those who plan to move (Golant, 1991). *Pathways* researchers have previously reported that moving to a CCRC does not reduce and may enhance social interaction among older adults (Erickson, Dempster-McClain, Whitlow, & Moen, 2000).

RELOCATION TO CONGREGATE FACILITIES

Congregate facilities include housing arrangements that are variously labeled as assisted living, residential care facilities, personal care homes, retirement homes, board-and-care homes, adult homes, continuing care retirement communities, parts of independent-living arrangements, and special residential sections of nursing homes (Schwarz & Brent, 1999). The Administration on Aging reported that, not including nursing homes, 2.4% of those 65 and older were living in congregate facilities, assisted-living, or board-and-care homes in 1990 (Administration on Aging, 1996). It is estimated that as many as 1 million older adults are living in a variety of housing circumstances referred to generally as assisted-living residences, but increasing numbers of older adults are expected to move to such supportive living environments in the future (Anikeef & Mueller, 1998; Speare, Avery & Lawton, 1991). In addition to those residing in assisted living, Feinberg (as cited in Anikeeff & Mueller, 1998) estimates some 750,000 older adults live in CCRCs and 500,000 live in congregate living communities.

Unfortunately, there is a dearth of research into why older adults relocate to congregate facilities. It is generally assumed that older adults move to these environments not out of choice but because of declines in health, social supports, or finances. Migration to a retirement community may meet the needs of two distinct groups. The first group includes those who are younger and healthier and are motivated by the amenities. The second group includes those who are older, less healthy, socially isolated, desire the support services retirement communities offer (Silverstein & Zablotsky, 1996) and want to reduce the need for home maintenance (Loomis, Sorece and Tyler, 1989). Other factors include limited mobility, inadequate public transportation, unexpected life events, and family concerns regarding physical and psychosocial well-being (Young, 1998).

A number of factors are likely to inhibit older adults from moving into congregate facilities. They include the preference for living in noncongregate housing, the cost, negative stereotypes associated with nursing homes that are applied to congregate housing, and the lack of awareness and knowledge of congregate housing options. For example, a study published in 1996 found that 60% of respondents 70 and older had never heard of CCRCs, about half had never heard of assisted-living or congregate housing, and less than one-quarter had visited such facilities (Harvard & Louis Harris and Associates, 1996).

CONTINUING CARE RETIREMENT COMMUNITIES

It is likely that the decision to move to a CCRC involves a series of choice points. None of the extant research differentiates among the decision to move out of one's primary residence, the decision to live in a CCRC (vs. another facility or with family), and the decision to choose a specific CCRC. Rather, previous research into reasons for moving to CCRCs has collected data from residents after they moved into a CCRC or from individuals on waiting lists, and they include people who may or may not ultimately move. Overall, the reasons identified in previous studies include the availability of long-term care (mainly medical services), the desire to remain independent, and the desire to avoid having to maintain a home or being a burden on family (mainly children).

For example, Kichen and Roche (1990) in a study of 422 residents living in 45 CCRCs around the nation found 72% of residents reported health care services as a very important reason for moving to a CCRC. Similar or higher percentages have been reported in other studies of CCRC residents or those on waiting lists (Cohen, Tell, Batten & Larson, 1988; Sheehan & Karasik, 1995; Sherwood, Ruchlin, Sherwood & Morris, 1997; Tell, Cohen, Larson & Batten, 1987). Sheehan and Karasik also found that married residents, when compared to nonmarried individuals, were more likely to cite guaranteed health care as very important. And Cohen and colleagues reported that many married residents indicated that they had moved to a CCRC to guarantee care for their spouses and to be near them during nursing home stays. Interestingly, Sherwood and colleagues (1997) found that a reason for moving to a CCRC given by a large majority of residents, access to needed services, was less often mentioned by those who had lived there longer, perhaps because they had begun to use such services.

The importance of the desire to remain independent as a reason for moving to a CCRC has been documented by several studies. Kichen and Roche (1990) report that three quarters of the residents of 45 CCRCs across the country indicated this aspect to be very important. Given the desire to remain independent, it is not surprising to find that avoiding being a burden on family also ranks high on the list of reasons for moving to a CCRC. Sherwood and colleagues (1997) reported that between 62 and 78% of residents in 19 CCRCs indicated this reason.

Finally, it is clear that other services matter as well. Sheehan and Karasik (1995) found that a wish to gain safety and security (43%), supplemental services (55%), and (another kind of independence perhaps) freedom from home upkeep and maintenance (83%) were also highly ranked as reasons for moving to a CCRC. Several researchers also found that protection against the potentially high costs of long-term care was an important CCRC relocation factor (Kichen & Roche, 1990; Tell, Cohen, Larson, & Batten, 1987). As noted earlier, reported reasons differed on the basis of demographic status. For example, younger respondents and those with more children and lower incomes were more likely to be concerned about finances and the family estate (Cohen, Tell, Batten, & Larson, 1988). Women and unmarried individuals were more apt to desire the security, planned social activities, and relief from loneliness offered by CCRCs (Sheehan and Karasik, 1995).

ATTITUDES TOWARD MOVING AMONG OLDER ADULTS

In addition to the reasons given by older individuals for relocating to congregate facilities, information about what they expect or anticipate doing in terms of future living arrangements is of interest and value to researchers and to planners and practitioners alike. Previous research has shown that measures of expectations are useful in estimating future behavior (Juster, 1997). Older adults who plan to move are 16 times more likely to actually move than are those who do not plan to move (Colsher & Wallace, 1990). Paradoxically, however, the majority of actual moves are made by older adults who do not plan to move (Colsher & Wallace, 1990). The large percentage of unplanned moves speaks to the prevailing desire to remain in established homes for as long as possible until unforeseen dependency forces the issue (Colsher & Wallace, 1990). People who *plan* to move tend to have more education and higher incomes. Those who actually move, however, have less education, have lower income, are physically dependent, and live alone. Johnson-Carroll, Brandt, and McFadden (1995) identify several factors that reduce the preference and propensity to move among pre-retirees. They include good health, looking forward to retirement, confidence in their maintenance skills, older age, living in a small house that is a detached single-family dwelling, having lived for many years in the same community, having definite tenure and structure preferences that would mimic their current structure (only perhaps smaller), and having definite plans about where to retire.

As noted earlier, a large majority of Americans prefers and expects to age in place. A 1990 AARP (1993) national survey reported that 85% of respondents 55 years old indicated that they never wanted to move, whereas approximately 70% of a national sample surveyed in 2000 indicated that they never plan to move (Harper & Bayer, 2000). Only one-quarter of those who did anticipate moving had a plan for their future living arrangements (Harper and Bayer, 2000). Aging in place may be a conscious choice or it may simply be a default living arrangement that results from a lack of planning (Dobkin, 1992). In addition, older adults can employ compensatory measures such as home modifications and supplemental care to remain in their homes when faced with physical and cognitive limitations. Harper and Bayer found that 70% of respondents in their survey of people age 55 years old and older who were permitted to adapt their environment to their needs had made one or more major home modifications. Assistance from others also supports the preference to age in place. Nearly 9.5 million Americans 50 and older receive supplemental care from family, friends, or home health care providers (Kassner & Bectel, 1998). Changing one's housing is obviously another strategy for effecting a favorable person-environment fit (Germain, 1994).

Moving in with family members is sometimes an intermediary step between independent living and moving to congregate housing. Most older adults, however, do not want to live in a family member's home (Harper & Bayer, 2000). A 1990 AARP (1993) survey found that only 17% of older respondents said they would consider moving in with a family member. In addition to seniors' desire to maintain independence, the changing family structure (fewer marriages, a higher divorce rate, having children later in life, having fewer or no children, and women having careers) can diminish the amount of support older adults receive from family and has dramatic implications for housing (U.S. Bureau of the Census, 1996). Thus it is possible that older adults will be increasingly likely to move to congregate or supportive housing alternatives because they are unable to rely upon their children for care.

Despite these trends, few researchers have investigated the attitudes and expectations older adults have about moving to congregate facilities. The findings of the *Pathways* study follow. First, we examine and compare the reasons given by older adults for moving into the CCRC or independent-living apartments in a facility that combines that housing option with assisted living. In each case we report the reasons given prior to moving. We also compare the moving plans of people living in a variety of residential settings and look at the likelihood older adults residing outside of housing facilities assign to the possibility of living in a range of housing options in the future.

FINDINGS OF THE *PATHWAYS* STUDY

RELOCATION TO THE CCRC AND INDEPENDENT-LIVING FACILITY

We examine data from 91 individuals who were part of the 1995 pilot study and who moved into the CCRC when it first opened (the CCRC founders) and data from 51 individuals who moved from the community between 1997–1998 and 1999–2000 into an independent-living facility (IL founders) that also has assisted living but not a nursing home. We report the findings of two questions about reasons for moving. The first asked What are the main reasons for your decision to move from your primary residence? The second asked What were the important considerations for you in looking for a new residence? The first asks for the general reasons that led respondents to move to the facility, and the other delves into the desired characteristics of their new residence. Both groups were asked these questions prospectively, before they moved, so the responses provide a unique insight into what residents of congregate-living facilities are thinking about and looking for as they plan to move. They also are among the first cohort of individuals moving into both of these new facilities and thus are termed *founders*.

Table 2.1 presents data on the percentage of respondents who select the various reasons for moving and the important factors each group considers in a new residence. The three most important reasons reported by CCRC founders for moving were to seek continuing care (85%); to be released from the burden of household upkeep and maintenance (53%); and to avoid becoming a burden on their families (44%). The respondent's current health and the respondent's spouse's current health (both 11%) were less frequently mentioned reasons for moving. Both the desire to obtain security in continuing care and to avoid becoming a burden on family involve anticipation of future needs. The release from household upkeep and maintenance could be viewed as a current need, a future need, or both. Considerably lower percentages of those who move into independent-liv-

TABLE 2.1 Reasons for Relocation and Important Considerations in a New Residence for CCRC Founders and Movers to Independent Living

	CCRC founders[a] (n = 91)	Independent living[b] (n = 51)
Reasons for relocation		
Size of residence	15.2	9.1
Upkeep and maintenance	52.7	24.2
Crime/safety	4.4	3.0
Death of spouse	2.2	6.1
Illness of spouse	11.0	9.1
Desire to be near family	4.4	9.1
Spouse wants to move	7.7	0.0
Family encouragement	3.3	0.0
Desire to live with peers	8.8	9.1
Loneliness	5.5	6.1
Illness	11.0	24.2
Avoid dependency on others	44.0	12.1
Future needs	84.6	60.6
Inability to get around	13.2	9.1
Considerations in new residence		
Location near relatives/friends	36.3	34.8
Proximity to recreational/cultural activities	31.9	34.8
Size/design of units	31.9	30.4
Personal security system	8.8	21.7
On-site medical/nursing services	60.4	17.4
Cost	18.7	26.1
On-site services/recreation	29.7	65.2
Kitchen facilities	19.8	26.1
Transportation	14.3	13.0
Decent place to live	23.1	30.4
Compatible people	31.9	26.1
Independence	36.3	17.4
Well-managed/quality staff	30.8	26.1
Reputation	35.2	50.0
Location	23.1	13.0
Maintenance free	35.2	26.1
Continuing care	71.4	39.1
Climate/geographical area	19.8	8.7
Family choice	1.1	4.3

[a] Data collected pre-move in 1995.
[b] Data collected pre-move in 1997.

ing facilities select these reasons (61% and 12%, respectively). Also of interest is the lower percentage of movers to independent-living facilities, as compared to CCRC founders, who select upkeep and maintenance as their reason (24% compared to 53%) and the higher percentage who select illness as their reason (24% compared to 11%).

Thus, the CCRC founders were much more likely to indicate concerns over upkeep and maintenance, dependency, and continuing care than were the IL founders. Interestingly, individuals moving into the independent-living facility that has less on-site health care and no skilled nursing facility were most likely to note illness as a reason for moving. Nonetheless, despite these differences, it is clear that the primary reasons for moving into these congregate facilities have to do with anticipating the need for future care, not being a burden on others, and not having to deal with the upkeep and maintenance of a residence.

Table 2.1 also reports on the most important considerations in selecting a new residence. As we can see, these reasons differ considerably from those given for moving in general. CCRC founders are again most likely to note continuing care (71%), but on-site medical and nursing services (60%) is a strong second. Both of these are far more likely to be identified as considerations than a third tier of factors, all of which were selected by about one third of the founders and include living in close proximity to family and friends (36%); a desire to remain independent (36%); the reputation of the facility (35%); freedom from maintenance (35%); living close to cultural activities, the size, design, or choice of living units, and living near compatible people (all 32%); the facility's reputation for being well-managed (31%); and on-site services and recreation (30%). These choices reflect concern with the nature of the facility (physical and operational) and social relationship and participation factors. Less than 20% of founders note cost, transportation, or climate.

The IL founders present another profile of what older adults look for in a congregate facility. Continuing care is no longer the consideration most likely to be selected (39%); more respondents select on-site services and recreation (65%). The perceived quality of the facility is more likely to be noted; "reputation" is selected by 50% and "decent place to live" by 30% of these movers. Social relationship and participation factors such as proximity to friends and to recreational and cultural opportunities and characteristics of the facility such as type of unit, cost, maintenance, and staff also emerge as factors for one quarter to one third of movers to the independent-living facility.

What can we say in general about the data shown in Table 2.1? First, we see that planning for future needs, dealing with the upkeep of a property, and avoiding dependency on others (or maintaining independence, if you will) stand out as the primary reasons for moving, regardless of the facility. These older movers like to plan ahead. Second, we do see a relationship between the facility type and the most important reasons given for moving there. While social relationships and facility characteristics are cited by all, those moving into the independent-living facility are much more likely to note services and recreation than are those moving into the continuing-care facility. This, in fact, reflects the differences between the two facilities. The independent-living facility does not have a skilled nursing home but does have a more structured program (and dedicated staff) for recreational services.

LOGISTIC REGRESSIONS

Logistic regressions, a statistical test used when the dependent variable is a categorical variable, were used to identify significant predictors of important considerations in moving. This was done for CCRC founders only, as the number (N) of IL founders was not large enough. In this analysis, independent variables are used to predict the likelihood of membership in one of the two dependent categories and are expressed as odds ratios. Multiple logistic regressions were estimated to see if reasons for moving or considerations in moving could be predicted by the demographic factors. Interaction terms were created for Marital Status times Age Cohort, Age Cohort times Perceived Health, and Marital Status times Perceived Health. These terms were also tested as predictors of reasons for moving in multiple logistic regressions. The findings are presented next.

Among CCRC founders, those with higher levels of education and whose spouses are in poor health are more likely to say that they would like to move because of their spouses' health. Respondents who rate their health as being poorer are more likely to state that their ability to get around is a reason to consider moving from their primary residence. Married women tend to mention their ability to get around as a consideration, whereas unmarried women did not mention this at all. Within the sample, 16% of married women indicate that either they had never learned to drive or do not currently drive. It is not unreasonable to assume that married women would be more dependent on their husbands for transportation whereas unmarried women would be much more independent in this regard.

An interaction of marital status and perceived health shows that married and unmarried women who report better health are more likely than married men to report the upkeep and maintenance of their home as a reason for relocating. This finding could reflect a couple of different factors. Married women might dependent on their husbands for household upkeep and have concerns about the future of home maintenance. Also, the unmarried women in our sample are significantly older than both the married women and the men, so unmarried women, even those in better health, may perceive themselves as being unable to continue with the upkeep and maintenance of their home. Age is not a significant factor in this portion of the analysis but it may have been significant had the sample size been larger.

For important considerations in a CCRC, odds ratios indicate that younger respondents (less than 77 years old) are 4.59 times more likely than older respondents to express a desire to move to a location that is close to cultural activities. Those who rate their health as being better are also more likely to mention that climate would be a factor in finding a new residence. Presumably, younger respondents and those who are in better health would be more active and interested in activities outside of the CCRC.

Finally, in the case of the independent living facility, we compare the reasons given prospectively for moving by those who subsequently did or did not move. Those who did not move to the facility were more likely than those who did move to report considering moving because of their own or the spouse's illness, while the movers to the independent-living facility were more likely to report that anticipating future needs was a reason for moving. Those who actually did move to the independent-living facility were more likely to report choosing the facility because of its location near relatives, friends, recreation, and culture and its on-site services. This suggests that those who actually moved saw the move as a proactive choice, one taken to minimize the impact of a future illness, whereas those who considered the facility but did not move were more concerned about what to do in a future crisis.

MOVING PLANS AND CHARACTERISTICS OF MOVERS

Pathways researchers also asked about moving plans and the likelihood that respondents would move into specific kinds of living arrangements. We look at the likelihood that individuals would move in several of the residential groupings in our study and compare the significant differences among individuals in the various moving-plan groups. We also report data for movers and nonmovers on the waiting list for the independent-living facility and look at the change in moving plans over a 2-year period.

TABLE 2.2 Descriptive Statistics for Four Subsamples by Moving Plans, Wave 1

Variable	Would not consider moving	Might consider moving	Currently considering moving	Significance
Community respondents (n = 455)	28.4%	58.7%	13.0%	
Age at interview	71.8 (8.1)	71.0 (7.1)	68.8 (6.7)	*
Female	54.3%	61.4%	74.6%	*
Education				
High school or less	36.4%	20.2%	23.7%	*
Some college or				
college degree	37.2%	41.9%	42.4%	
Graduate school	26.4%	37.8%	33.9%	
Household composition				
Married, living				
with spouse	65.1%	66.3%	45.8%	*
Lives with				
non-spouse	10.9%	8.2%	13.6%	
Lives alone	24.0%	25.5%	40.7%	
Has a local child	65.1%	62.2%	40.7%	**
Local family				
(spouse or child)	85.3%	88.8%	66.1%	***
New facility waiting list (n = 101)	5.9%	38.6%	55.4%	
Household composition				
Married, living				
with spouse	33.3%	76.9%	50.0%	**
Lives with				
non-spouse	16.7%	0%	1.8%	
Lives alone	50.0%	23.1%	48.2%	
Perceived health	6.8 (1.7)	7.9 (1.4)	7.1 (1.9)	*
Senior housing residents (n = 143) (No significant differences)	58.0%	37.8%	4.2%	
CCRC residents (n = 55)	80.0%	20.0%	0%	
Local family				
(spouse or child)	56.8%	90.9%		*

Source: Pathways to Life Quality, 1998
+ p < .10; * p < .05; ** p < .01; *** p < .001.

Table 2.2 shows responses for three moving categories (would not consider, might consider, and currently considering) based on four subsamples of the data: nonfacility residents, those on the independent-living waiting list, those currently living in senior housing but not in the CCRC, and those living in the CCRC. The question was asked only of CCRC residents who had moved in after the facility first opened; it is a different group from the one reported on in Table 2.1. The CCRC residents are treated as a separate category because it is assumed they do not plan to move, given that the main reason they moved in the first place was for so they could have life-long care. As expected, this group is most likely *not* to consider moving (80%) whereas those on the waiting list are most likely to be currently considering moving (55%). No CCRC residents and only a very few other senior housing residents are currently thinking of moving. Community residents, on the other hand, fall in between the other groups. Almost three fifths of them indicate they might consider moving and 13% say they are currently doing so.

Table 2.2 also shows data comparing these categories on the basis of a variety of independent variables. A number of these variables differentiate the moving plans of community respondents and those on the waiting list for the independent-living facility, but no variables are related to moving plans for senior-housing residents, and only one (having a spouse or child who lives locally) is related to plans for CCRC residents. For community residents, those currently considering moving are younger; more likely to be female; less likely to be married and living with the spouse; less likely to have family or a child living locally; and more likely to have had a high school education or less. People on the independent-living facility's waiting list who would not consider moving report the lowest perceived health score, on average, and are less likely to be married and living with the spouse.

Not reported in Table 2.2 are findings on changes in moving plans between 1997 and 1999. Overall, plans are fairly stable, with 63% reporting the same likelihood of moving; 20% are less likely and 17% more likely to move or to consider moving. Most of those who had moved (75%), however, thought it less likely that they would move again. Life course and decision-making theories suggest that individuals are continually evaluating the suitability of their current housing, so we thought that changes in some life circumstances would be associated with changes in moving plans. In particular, we hypothesized that widowhood, health declines, and children moving into or away from the local area would affect respondents' moving plans. Although recent widows not in senior housing are some-what more likely to consider moving, health declines and changes in children's proximity are not associated with changes in moving plans. It may be that relatively small health declines such as those seen over the 2-year interval are not enough to overcome factors such as attachment to place and ties to the community.

Last, only in the case of those moving to the independent-living facility do we have data, at this point in the study, that allows us to compare the characteristics of those on the waiting list who moved versus those who did not move during the 2-year period. Those who moved were less likely to have high incomes ($60,000 or more) or to live in a single-family home and were more likely to live alone, suggesting that those with more financial and social resources can rely on private residence options for a longer time. The groups did not differ on a number of other characteristics, including home satisfaction, length of residence, space, privacy, and social integration.

ANTICIPATED LIVING ARRANGEMENTS

Finally, we examine the types of living arrangements older adults in the community expect to experience in the future. Respondents were asked to indicate on a scale of 0 to 100 the likelihood that they would live in particular living arrangements in the future. In 1997, respondents were given six options, but because two were selected by a very small percentage of the sample, only four options were presented in 1999. As the data in Table 2.3 show, aging in place and making major modifications to one's current residence and given the highest likelihood, on average (71% and 61%, respectively, in 1997).

These numbers are comparable to those from 1999, with 71% giving the highest likelihood to staying without modifications. However, remaining with modifications dropped to 51%. Respondents view a move to a retirement community as a significant possibility, rating it as a one in three chance at both interviews. Many respondents added comments to their ratings, the majority saying that moving to a retirement community was a last resort, an option to be considered only if they couldn't stay in their homes with assistance from caregivers. Those who rated moving to a retirement community high often mentioned that they were in the process of looking into retirement communities or had placed their names on one or more waiting lists. Those who rated the option very low made some of the following comments:

TABLE 2.3 Likelihood Ratings for Future Living Arrangements of the Random Community

Living Arrangement	1997		1999	
	Mean	SD	Mean	SD
Age in place (no major modifications)	71%	32	71%	34
Age in place (with modifications)	61%	37	51%	41
Age in place (with assistance)	—	—	61%	36
Retirement community	32%	32	33%	32
Move in with family	16%	27	10%	22
Shared household	9%	19	—	—
Removable home	16%	27	—	—
Move closer to family	—	—	24%	32
Move to smaller home	—	—	27%	33

Sample (n = 346).

"No, because the rooms are cramped and it's too claustrophobic for my husband. For me, there is a lack of privacy and personal space."
"Eventually, if I lose my mind."
"Maybe someday when I'm old."

Moving in with family members is the least appealing option for our respondents and the idea often elicited strong responses. When asked about moving in with family, one respondent was quick to say, "I grew up with three grandmothers in a large house. I learned that no house is big enough for more than one grown woman." Other comments include:

"That's a no-no. They have their ideas for family and we have ours. Those things would just clash."
"Wouldn't want it, no way."
"One son offered, but I think that it would be a disaster."
"They've moved in here!"

Our data show that the majority of community-dwelling elders expect to remain in their current homes. Some expect to make modifications and some don't. If they need care, they expect to get it at home. Following them over time will allow us to determine if they indeed can fulfill these expectations.

IMPLICATIONS FOR RESEARCH, POLICY, AND PRACTICE

The *Pathways* findings expand the existing knowledge base concerning housing preferences and reasons for moving of older adults. Our data on reasons for moving to a CCRC reinforce the importance of the availability of long-term care services and other services such as home maintenance and upkeep and the desire to avoid dependency on others noted by other researchers. But they also suggest that these reasons vary according to the type of housing involved. Study participants who moved to independent-living facilities were less likely to identify these reasons. Additional factors emerge, such as the facility's characteristics (management quality and housing characteristics), location and proximity to community activities, and proximity to relatives and friends. Again, we see differences based on the type of facility. Our findings suggest caution; researchers should consider the nature of the destination when attempting to generalize from research about reasons for moving by older adults. The reasons will be likely to vary depending on the nature of the housing moved to. Furthermore, small differences in the questions about reasons for relocation can elicit very different responses.

We also have generated findings of note about expectations and preferences when moving. Again, our research stresses the importance of the housing environment—in this case, whether or not an older person lives in a facility and the type of facility it is. The older adults in our study who have recently moved to a CCRC express no intention of and little interest in moving, whereas those living in other congregate facilities and, especially, in the community are much more likely to consider moving. Given the strong preference of older adults to age in place, it is interesting to note that almost 60% of our sample living in the community indicated they might consider moving and 13% were actively considering doing so. The *Pathways* study is one of the few, to our knowledge, that asks about the type of living arrangements older adults anticipate experiencing in the future. Here we found the well-documented expectation of aging in place, but (for community-dwelling elders, at least) a fairly high probability of making major home modifications. And despite the plethora of studies that have reported the strong preference for and prevalence of familial caregiving, respondents in our study state that the likelihood of living in a retirement community is more than two and one half times greater than moving in with family.

It is clear that far too little data have been collected on the relocation preferences and behavior of older adults. The *Pathways* study provides information for one community and is not necessarily generalizable to the older population nationwide. More data are needed concerning older adults' expectations about moving in general and about the particular types of housing arrangements they desire. Our study looks at the reasons people voluntarily relocate and provides a comparison of movers to a congregate facility and nonmovers among those who had previously indicated an interest in moving. Much more research is needed into the circumstances that lead older adults to move from a private dwelling to a congregate community. When and how is this decision made, and what circumstances are associated with the decision to move as opposed to making home modifications or seeking additional services from informal or formal supports?

Our findings have several implications for policy makers. First, our findings suggest a relatively low expectation that older adults will move in with a family member. While this desire for "intimacy at a distance" with adult children is not surprising, it reinforces the need for policy makers to develop, implement, and support a long-term care policy that provides multiple housing options for older adults. Despite the growth of the assisted living industry in the United States, current policy is predicated primarily on the concept that older people have three options when long-term care needs emerge: stay at home, move in with a family member, or move to a nursing home. It is important to recognize that housing should be a core part of long-term care planning and policy. Second, the interest in home modifications as a way of facilitating aging in place suggests the need for education about the types, costs, and effectiveness of these modifications. Very few public dollars are currently available for housing modification because most public housing programs are aimed at new construction. The housing industry, until recently, has seen little financial incentive in home rehabilitation or modification. This is a policy issue that might be addressed by public-private partnerships. Third, census data on older adults reveal that they are less likely to move than younger adults, and most of the focus given to older adult migration is on in migration to Sunbelt states and out migration from the Snowbelt states and the Midwest. Our data show older people do consider other housing options. Because expectations are likely predictors of future housing moves, awareness of the kinds of housing options older adults consider and the changes in them over time will help planners develop realistic and effective housing policies that will meet future needs.

Finally, the *Pathways* findings on relocation are instructive for practitioners in several areas, such as care management, home care, information and referral coordination, and public- private partnerships and coalitions. The first finding is, again, that respondents see making major home modifications as being quite likely in the future. This suggests a potential demand for these kinds of services and the resources to pay for them at the local level. Information and referral programs as well as education to assist older adults in making better informed decisions about these products would be appropriate. It also means that practitioners must develop expertise in assessing need and developing programs in this area. In addition, resources will be needed for low-income seniors if the most vulnerable are to be adequately served. Practitioners can be important advocates for such resources, but being a good advocate will require high-quality data on need, costs of services, and the efficacy of home modifications compared with other programs. The interest shown in retirement communities also suggests the need for practitioners to develop an understanding of these housing options. Similarly, the relatively high percentage of respondents indicating they would consider moving suggests the need for practitioners to have more information about the impact of moving on older individuals, their families, and their communities.

SUMMARY AND CONCLUSIONS

This chapter provides an overview of what we know about the relocation behavior of older adults and presents findings from the *Pathways* study concerning the reasons for moving and the expectation of doing so. We find that the reasons for moving vary with the housing type. Underlying the moving by older people into a CCRC, according to the *Pathways* study, are the desires to remain independent, to avoid the need to perform upkeep and maintenance, and to avoid being a burden on family. Movers to independent-living facilities also relocate in anticipation of meeting future needs, but look for somewhat different features in their new residential setting.

Our data reveal that older adults are more likely to be considering or planning a move than was previously thought. Indeed, only 3 of 10 respondents living outside of congregate settings would not consider moving. While aging in place is the most likely housing future seen by older adults living outside of congregate settings, the likelihood of making major home modifications is fairly high. Moving in with family members is given a very low probability, but receiving assistance from them is seen as being more likely and is given about the same probability as moving to a retirement community.

These findings suggest that researchers, policy makers, and practitioners should look more closely at the reasons for moving and at the current and future housing plans of older adults. The older adults themselves are likely to experience the need for relocation and must become better informed consumers of housing options. The decision to relocate is multifaceted and involves factors related to the current and anticipated states of health and well-being of self and partner, the characteristics of the housing itself, the availability of social support, and the availability of housing and community amenities and resources. A better understanding of these factors and why and where older people decide to move will assist older adults and their families make more appropriate housing decisions and will assist governments, communities, and the housing industry better plan for the needs of an aging population.

REFERENCES

Administration on Aging. (1996). *The road to an aging policy for the 21st century.* 1995 White House Conference on Aging. Washington, DC: Author.

American Association of Retired People. (1993). *Understanding senior housing for the 1990s.* Washington, DC: Author.

American Association of Retired People. (1996, September). *Understanding senior housing: Into the next century.* Washington, DC: Author.

Anikeeff, M. A., & Mueller, G. R. (Eds.). (1998). *Senior housing.* Boston: Kluwer Academic.

Choi, N. G. (1996). Older persons who move: Reasons and health consequences. *Journal of Applied Gerontology, 15*(3), 325–344.

Clark, W. A., & Davies, S. (1990). Elderly mobility and mobility outcomes: Households in the later stages of the life course. *Research on Aging, 12*(4), 430–462.

Cohen, M., Tell, E., Batten, H., & Larson, M. (1988). Attitudes toward joining continuing care retirement communities. *The Gerontologist, 28*(5), 637–643.

Colsher, P. L., & Wallace, R. B. (1990). Health and social antecedents of relocation in rural elderly persons. *Journal of Gerontology, 45*(1), S32–S38.

Dobkin, L. (1992, Spring). If you build it, they may not come. *Generations, 16,* 31–32.

Erickson, M. A., Dempster-McClain, D., Whitlow, C., & Moen, P. (2000). Social integration and the move to a continuing care retirement community. In K. Pillemer, P. Moen, E. Wethington, & N. Glasgow (Eds.), *Social integration in the second half of life* (pp. 211–227). Baltimore: Johns Hopkins University.

Ferraro, K. F. (1983). Health consequences of relocation among the aged in the community. *Journal of Gerontology, 38*(1), 90–96.

Flynn, C. B., Longino, C. F., Jr., Wiseman, R. F., & Biggar, J. C. (1985). Redistribution of America's older population: Major national migration patterns for three census decades, 1960–1980. *The Gerontologist, 25*(3), 292–296.

Germain, C. B. (1994). Using an ecological perspective. In J. Rothman (Ed.), *Practice with highly vulnerable clients* (pp. 39–55). Englewood Cliffs, NJ: Prentice-Hall.

Golant, S. M. (1991). Matching congregate housing settings with a diverse elderly population: Research and theoretical considerations. *Journal of Housing for the Elderly, 9*(1–2), 21–38.

Haas, W. H., III, & Serow, W. J. (1993). Amenity retirement migration process: A model and preliminary evidence. *The Gerontologist, 33*(2), 212–220.

Harper, L., & Bayer, A-H. (2000). *Fixing to stay: A national survey of housing and home modification issues.* Washington, DC: AARP.

Harvard School of Public Health and Louis Harris and Associates. (1996). *Long-term care awareness survey.* Cambridge: Harvard University.

Johnson-Carroll, K. J. A., Brandt, J. A., & McFadden, J. R. (1995). Factors that influence pre-retirees' propensity to move at retirement. *Journal of Housing for the Elderly, 11*(2), 85–105.

Juster, F. T. (1997). On the measurement of expectations, uncertainty, and preferences. *Journal of Gerontology: Social Sciences, 52B*(5), S237–S239.

Kassner, E., & Bectel, R. W. (1998). *Midlife and older Americans with disabilities: Who gets help?* Washington, DC: AARP.

Kichen, J., & Roche, J. (1990). Life care resident preferences: A survey of the decision-making process to enter a CCRC. In R. D. Chellis & P. J. Grayson (Eds.), *Life care: A long-term solution?* (pp. 49–60). Lexington, MA: Lexington.

Lee, E. (1966). A theory of migration. *Demography, 3*(1), 47–57.

Litwak, E., & Longino, C. F. (1987). Migration patterns among the elderly: A developmental perspective. *The Gerontologist, 27*(3), 266–272.

Longino, C. F. (1990). Geographical distribution and migration. In R. H. Binstock & L. K. Geroge (Eds.), *Handbook of aging and the social sciences* (pp. 45–63). San Diego, CA: Academic.

Longino, C. F., Jr., & Fox, R. A. (Eds). (1995). *Retirement migration in America.* Houston, TX: Vacation Publications.

Longino, C. F., Jr., Jackson, D. J., Zimmerman, R. S., & Bradsher, J. E. (1991). The second move: Health and geographic mobility. *Journals of Gerontology: Social Sciences, 46*(4), S218–S224.

Loomis, L. M., Sorce, P., & Tyler, P. R. (1989). Lifestyle analysis of healthy retirees and their interest in moving to a retirement community. *Journal of Housing for the Elderly, 5*(2), 19–35.

Miller, M. E., Longino, C. F., Jr., Anderson, R. T., James, M. K., & Worley, A. S. (1999). Functional status, assistance, and the risk of a community-based move. *The Gerontologist, 39*(2), 187–200.

Mutchler, J. E., & Burr, J. A. (1991). A longitudinal analysis of household and non-household living arrangements in later life. *Demography, 28*(3), 375–390.

Pastalan, L. A. (Ed.). (1995). *Housing decisions for the elderly: To move or not to move.* Binghamton, NY: Haworth.

Pynoos, J., & Golant, S. (1996). Housing and living arrangements for the elderly. In R. H. Binstock & L. K. Gerorge (Eds.), *Handbook of aging and the social sciences* (4th ed., pp. 303–324). New York: Academic.

Pynoos, J., & Liebig, P. (1995). *Housing frail elders: International policies, perspectives, and prospects.* Baltimore: Johns Hopkins University.

Rogers, A. (1988). Age patterns of elderly migration: An international comparison. *Demography, 25*(3), 355–370.

Scheidt, R. J., & Windley, P. G. (Eds). (1998). *Environment and aging theory: A focus on housing.* Westport, CT: Greenwood.

Schwarz B., & Brent R. (Eds.). (1999). *Aging, autonomy, and architecture: Advances in assisted living.* Baltimore: Johns Hopkins University.

Sheehan, N., & Karasik, R. (1995). The decision to move to a continuing care retirement community. *Journal of Housing for the Elderly, 11*(2), 107–122.

Sherwood, S., Ruchlin, H., Sherwood, C., & Morris, S. (1997). *Continuing care retirement communities.* Baltimore: Johns Hopkins University.

Silverstein, M., & Zablotsky, D. L. (1996). Health and social precursors of later life retirement-community migration. *Journals of Gerontology: Series B: Psychological Sciences and Social Sciences, 51B*(3), S150–S156.

Sommers, D. G., & Rowell, K. R. (1992). Factors differentiating elderly residential movers and nonmovers: A longitudinal analysis. *Population Research and Policy Reviews, 11*(3), 249–262.

Speare, A., Jr., Avery R., & Lawton, L. (1991). Disability, residential mobility, and changes in living arrangements. *Journals of Gerontology: Social Sciences, 46*(3), S133–S142.

Tell, E., Cohen, M., Larson, M., & Batten, H. (1987). Assessing the elderly's preferences for lifecare retirement options. *The Gerontologist, 27*(4), 503–509.

Thomasma, M., Yeaworth, R. C., & McCabe, B. W. (1990). Moving day: Relocation and anxiety in institutionalized elderly. *Journal of Gerontological Nursing, 16*(7), 18–25.

Thorson, J. A. (1988). Relocation of the elderly: Some implications from the research. *Gerontology Review, 1*(1), 28–36.

U.S. Bureau of the Census. (1996). *65+ in the United States* (P23-190). Washington, DC: U.S.G.P.O.

U.S. Department of Commerce. (1998). *Seasonality of moves and duration of residence* (Series P70, No. 66). Washington, DC: K. A. Hansen.

Young, H. M. (1998). Moving to congregate housing: The last chosen home. *Journal of Aging Studies, 12*(2), 149–165.

CHAPTER 3

Housing Satisfaction: Design Lessons from the Community

Paul E. Eshelman, Gary W. Evans, and Shinobu Utamura

R esearch on residential relocation for older adults (see chapter 2) is complemented by research examining the places left behind after relocation. These residences of varying types and qualities scattered throughout communities are the places where the vast majority of older adults live and expect to age. Although preferences and expectations for aging in place can be explained in part by resistance to the change and decline inevitable in the aging process, people prefer and expect their housing to satisfy basic needs. Part of the push described in chapter 2 as precipitating relocation among the elderly includes upkeep and maintenance and future needs. Thus, a critical leverage point for prolonging aging in place is a better understanding of the role of the design characteristics that influence residential satisfaction among the elderly who still reside in the community.

Research on aging and the environment has focused more on elderly facility residents than on older community residents. As a result, relatively little research has examined the great majority of older adults who live independently in the community (Carp, 1987). Research that has targeted this population and investigated dwelling features that contribute to housing satisfaction has yielded discontinuous results that offer only fragmented design guidance. This chapter examines how the design features of residential units are related to residential satisfaction among elderly community members in the *Pathways to Life Quality* study. Reflection on this assessment results in a taxonomy for structuring subsequent studies of older adults' housing satisfaction. By linking behavioral principles and design decisions, the taxonomy identifies the design concepts to be used when modifying existing dwellings or creating new housing units for older adults choosing to remain in the community.

HOUSING SATISFACTION

Assessments of housing satisfaction have examined the predictive capability of environmental features on scales ranging from microenvironmental such as the hardware in the dwelling to macroenvironmental such as aspects of the neighborhood. Those features shown to be most powerful variables in self-report research operate at the macro scale of neighborhood or community. Jirovec, Jirovec, & Bosse (1984) reported that neighborhood satisfaction accounts for 92% of the variance in prediction of housing satisfaction. This finding is paralleled by Toseland and Rasch (1978) in their study of older persons' satisfaction with their community. A key finding was that subject satisfaction with individual dwelling units explained only a small amount (4.9%) of the total variance. When Lawton, Nahemow, and Teaff first reported their study of the characteristics of federally assisted housing environments and neighborhoods (1975), they found that neighborhood characteristics were highly related to housing satisfaction. Lawton and Nahemow went on in a subsequent study to speculate that a statistically significant dwelling variable, "ease of being visited," is "a proxy for judgment of neighborhood safety, centrality of location, or transportation access, rather than being related to building or dwelling-unit design." (1979, p. 11) These findings identify the importance of being mindful of the role of safe, supportive neighborhoods in enabling elderly residents to feel satisfied with their housing (Jirovec et al., 1984).

Although these studies suggest that microenvironmental features such as interior design features of the dwelling might be relatively unimportant in their contribution to residential satisfaction, such a conclusion is probably incorrect for several reasons. First, when macroenvironmental variables—for example, neighborhood satisfaction—are statistically controlled, dwelling-unit features remain significant predictors of housing satisfaction. Jirovec and colleagues (1984), when they excluded neighborhood satisfaction from their analysis, found that characteristics of individual dwellings explained 40% of the variance in subjects' housing satisfaction. Second, several of the previous studies of residential satisfaction defined satisfaction in such general or vague terms that it is not at all clear what respondents were evaluating (Golant, 1982; Toseland & Rasch, 1978).

Moreover, the plausible contribution of personal characteristics (e.g., income, personality) to the apparent linkages between neighborhood quality and residential satisfaction were not properly dealt with in previous studies. Third, all of these studies rely strictly on self-report measures for environmental assessments and for residential satisfaction. This raises serious concerns about the construct validity of the neighborhood environment index as well as about inflated covariation due to shared method.

A number of other studies support the conclusion that features at the scale of the individual dwelling explain significant variance in housing satisfaction (Christensen & Carp, 1987; Lawton, 1980b; Lawton & Nahemow, 1979; Zhu & Shelton, 1996). The challenge is to weave the findings of these and other studies together to provide coherent directives for the design of residential units for older adults. A number of inconsistencies or incomplete interpretations in the findings contribute to this challenge.

Some findings are at odds with obvious environmental needs of elderly residents. An example is the conclusion that the "majority of elderly homeowners were highly satisfied with their residences, even though their housing has deficiencies" (Zhu & Shelton, 1996, p. 30). A related example is that the absence of mobility supports needed by many older adults contributed to housing dissatisfaction (Lawton & Nahemow, 1979). These examples parallel the finding reported in chapter 2 that "those moving into independent-living facilities are much more likely to note services and recreation than are those moving into continuing care facilities" as a reason to move. A plausible explanation for the findings in these examples is that they reflect a human urge to deny the physical and mental decline that is fundamental to the aging process. Irrespective of the explanations, the challenge is to interpret the findings concerning housing satisfaction within a context of documented behavioral and emotional needs of the elderly.

Some findings justify an incomplete definition of good housing—the mere elimination of deficiencies. Deficient housing clearly prevails among the elderly living in the community. For those with sufficient means to move, household upkeep and maintenance are reported to be important reasons for moving. As documented in chapter 2, 53% of individuals who moved into the continuing care retirement community (CCRC) and 24% of those who moved into independent-living facilities reported household upkeep and maintenance to be important reasons for moving). Those who do not have the means to move—people on limited income with steadily rising housing costs—are forced to spend money needed for home maintenance on more immediate needs, thus sacrificing housing quality (Zhu

& Shelton, 1996). It is no wonder that housing satisfaction studies tend to use housing deficits as the independent variable (Struyk, 1977; Struyk & Turner, 1984; Weicher, 1986). What these studies may be finding, though, is that the residents surveyed were simply voicing an absence of dissatisfaction with deficient housing and not true satisfaction. Moreover as pointed out earlier, many measures of housing satisfaction are sufficiently general or vague that it is often difficult to know how elderly respondents interpret the index. Turning a blind eye toward the reality of a situation parallels the resistance to reminders of bodily deterioration with aging observed by Lawton and Nahemow (1979) in their finding of dissatisfaction with the presence of handrails in bathrooms. However salient housing deficits and prosthetic features may be, full understanding of housing satisfaction can not be achieved through studies that concentrate only on elimination of negative aspects of housing.

Still other findings do not represent the total reality of the housing experience of older adults living independently in the community. This reality has been described in terms of two variable categories: function and meaning (Eshelman & Evans, 2002). The study examined the relative contribution of two categories of interior features—functional features that respond to lower level human needs (Maslow, 1962) and features with personal meaning that address higher level needs of belonging and esteem (Maslow, 1962)—as predictors of place attachment and self-esteem for new retirement community residents housed in independent-living apartments or cottages. The key finding was that for both place attachment and self-esteem, significantly more variance is accounted for by adding meaning variables to function variables. Alternatively stated, unless spaces are functional, older adults cannot begin to feel attached to their place of residence and begin to feel good about themselves. Once functional needs are met, place attachment and self-esteem are elevated by interior features—preferred materials, finishes, and details—that have personal meaning and that support personalization.

The current literature on aging and the built environment almost exclusively addresses the function category. This appears to be the case in studies of older adults' housing satisfaction (Christensen & Carp, 1987; Lawton, 1980; Lawton & Nahemow, 1979; Zhu & Shelton, 1996). A few studies do, however, reach into the meaning side of the housing experience, addressing issues of aesthetics (Butterfield & Weidemann, 1987; Christensen et al., 1992; Christensen & Carp, 1987), familiarity (Jirovec et al., 1984; Zavotka & Teaford, 1997); and personalization (Butterfield & Weidemann,

1987; Eshelman & Evans, 2002). Others have proposed taxonomies that broaden the scope of the residential experience. A good example is Regnier's 12 design-behavior principles: privacy; social interactions; control/ choice/autonomy; orientation/way finding; safety/security; accessibility and functioning; stimulation/challenge; sensory aspects; familiarity; aesthetics/appearance; personalization; and adaptability (1994, pp. 44–46). These principles, in combination with consideration of cost (Zhu & Shelton, 1996), condition of building and utility systems, and structural integrity (Christensen, Carp, Cranze, & Wiley, 1992) could offer a more complete description of the residential experience.

Findings that fail to recognize individual differences among elderly community residents add to the challenge. As Bell, Fisher, Baum, & Greene (1996) have pointed out, there probably is no other cohort of the population with such a broad diversity of individual problems and needs, and these individual differences increase with age (Kelly, 1955). Differences in physical health, cognitive competency, behavior patterns established over a lifetime, social roles, preferred activities, and environmental preferences all add up to a subtly defined need for great environmental diversity in housing. Providing this level of environmental diversity is expensive (Lawton, 1980a), and can drive design efforts toward standardization in planned housing. It is important for housing satisfaction research to help resist the forces that drive standardization. Information about the amount of diversity that must be accommodated will lead to innovative thinking by designers.

Findings that fail to recognize the number and variety of decisions that are made in the design of housing hamper the identification of clear design directives. Thinking just in terms of dwellings' interiors, at least six categories of design decisions can be seen. The first, using the terminology of the designer, is to define the space. This entails decisions about square footage, ceiling heights, spatial volume, and spatial proportions with the intent of accommodating the anticipated activities of the occupant. Related spatial decisions involve defining the degree of enclosure or openness through handling of the enclosing planes and openings such as doorways and windows. Additional consideration must be given to relationships among adjoining spaces through attention to lines of sight and paths of circulation. Ideally, design decisions about adjacencies also incorporate concerns about privacy and the ability to regulate social interaction (Altman, 1975). Human needs for social interaction are dynamic, ranging across a continuum from solitude to group interaction. The provision of space that supports this continuum as well as thoughtfulness about the relative positioning of social spaces (e.g., spatial hierarchy ranging from public to private (Evans & McCoy, 1998) can facilitate privacy.

Our second category of interior design decisions involve features that are built in, such as bookshelves, cabinets, window seating, and banquette seating. These features are important in their capacity to maximize space efficiency, space-use flexibility, storage, and support for personalization, and in their capacity to minimize the total amount of floor space to be constructed. The third category is hardware selection, based on aesthetics as well as function of knobs, handles, railings, and fixtures. Ergonomic considerations are critical here, particularly for an aging population.

A fourth category calls for decisions about materials and finishes that affect ease of maintenance, usability, aesthetic quality, and feelings of hominess. Considerations of safety are also very important in selecting materials and finishes for an elderly population. The fifth category is furniture. Although this category typically is in the hands of the resident, the interior designer influences furniture decisions through the placement and arrangement opportunities that are created when the designer makes spatial decisions. Evidence indicates that neither designers nor the elderly are particularly accurate in their judgments about the role of such interior design features and safety. The sixth category is lighting. This category includes determining light levels, balancing the contributions of natural and artificial light, and selecting and placing fixtures. It is also important to consider the role of visual access. A good view can allow for vicarious as well as direct control within a neighborhood social setting; it may help to deter crime by allowing visual surveillance, and it can offer potentially restorative experiences by allowing sight of nearby nature (Evans & McCoy, 1998).

It is important to note that defining these six categories of design does not imply that decisions are made categorically. In fact, decisions typically are made in concert with attention to interrelationships. For example, lighting decisions are inseparable from spatial decisions about openings and the flow of natural light into a space. And color is by no means relegated only to the category of materials and finishes. Perception of color is affected by lighting, spatial volume, and the proximity of different colors. Also, prosthetic decisions cross into all of the categories—lighting decisions require consideration of visual access to items displayed in built-in cabinets; hardware decisions require consideration of the ergonomics of door handles, handrails, and grab bars; and material decisions require consideration of the rolling resistance of flooring materials so wheelchairs can operate smoothly.

Research into housing satisfaction among elderly community members would be most useful to designers if findings were linked to categories of design decisions.

PRESENT STUDY

In the *Pathways to Life Quality* study, 29 housing features were used as predictors of housing satisfaction by regression analyses. Of these, the first 20 relate to function. The remaining 9 deal with aesthetics and meaning. It is to be noted that 25 of these 29 items are based upon evaluations of the interior environments by trained raters. The remaining 4 items are based on the replies of the respondents. Table 3.1 lists the 29 items and illustrates how they can be grouped in terms of the six categories of design decisions.

The dependent variable in this study, overall housing satisfaction, was measured using a 29-item scale (e.g., this is a comfortable living unit; I don't like living here; this place is close to my ideal living environment; my home has adequate storage; the space in my home is adequate for sleeping) that has a reliability coefficient of a = .84. Controlling for income and negative affect, two variables that have an impact on subjective housing satisfaction, the results of regression of housing features on housing satisfaction show that 31% of the variance in housing satisfaction of community adults is explained by overall design features: $\Delta R^2 = .31$, $F(31, 496) = 7.24$, $p < .0001$. Negative affectivity is the tendency to focus on the more negative aspects of life, and it can distort subjective evaluations. By statistically controlling for this personality characteristic, a more sensitive index is achieved (Watson & Pennebaker, 1989).

When the 29 housing features were considered simultaneously, 8 items listed in Table 3.2 emerged as significant and independent predictors of housing satisfaction.

Given the wide degree of heterogeneity of the aging population in the United States (Bell et al., 1996; Kelly, 1955), it is also important to examine whether interior design features that influence overall housing satisfaction interact with personal characteristics of the elderly. By *interact*, we mean whether the effects of specific design variables on satisfaction vary or are moderated by personal characteristics. Do men and women respond similarly in terms of satisfaction to various design characteristics of housing? Are elderly with varying degrees of physical health affected similarly? Does how old one is affect reaction to these various features?

TABLE 3.1 Relationship Between Categories of Design Decisions and Housing Feature Items

design decisions
about spatial volume, proportions, and connections among spaces
  about custom-built features
    about hardware
      about surface treatments—materials, finishes, color
        about furniture and equipment
          about lighting

spatial volume, proportions, connections	custom-built features	hardware	surface treatments—materials, finishes, color	furniture and equipment	lighting	Interview Items
X						1. Enter residence from outside without using stairs?
X						2. Ramps at street level?
X						3. Exterior door wide enough for a wheelchair?
X						4. Do you have to climb stairs within your home or apartment to get to any area of your home that you use every day?
X						5. Any unexpected floor-level changes?
					X	6. Main entrance well lighted?
					X	7. Hallways well lighted?
					X	8. Stairways well lighted?
					X	9. Light over sink or mirror?
					X	10. Bathing area well lighted?
					X	11. Task lighting over activity areas?
X						12. Open counter space sufficient to prepare a meal?
	X					13. Do you need a stool or ladder to use any cabinets or storage areas in your home?
	X					14. Are there any storage areas that are too close to the ground for you to reach easily?
X	X	X				15. Modifications for interior wheelchair use?
		X				16. Handrails in the main hallway?
		X				17. Handrails/safety bars in shower or tub?
		X				18. Grab bars near toilet?
				X		19. Seat in shower?
			X			20. Nonslip areas in bathroom?
			X		X	21. Do you consider your room/apartment/house colorful or subdued?
			X		X	22. During the day, do you consider your room/apartment/house bright or dark?
	X					23. Wood trim?
	X					24. Custom cabinetry?
	X					25. Fireplace or wood stove?
	X					26. Window seat?
	X					27. Deep windowsills for plants?
X				X		28. Easy to find space to arrange valued possessions that have personal meaning—such as books, artwork, and furniture?
				X	X	29. Personal objects and displays are lit in a way that allows me to see them well.

TABLE 3.2 Regression of Housing Features on Housing Satisfaction

Variable	b	SE	ß
Space for valued possessions	4.87***	.77	.28
Personal objects lit	3.88***	.85	.20
Task lighting	2.59**	1.03	.10
Deep window sills for plants	− 2.50*	1.08	−.10
Safety bars in tub	2.45*	1.15	.10
Custom cabinetry	2.17*	1.12	.08
Main entrance well lighted	6.28*	2.84	.09
Window seats	3.09*	1.53	.08

b = unstandardized regression coefficient;
ß = standardized regression coefficient;
SE = standard error;
n = 527;
R^2 = .31;
*$p < .05$; **$p < .01$; ***$p < .001$.

In order to address these questions, we conducted a second set of regression analyses to supplement the overall, main effects described earlier. For all of the original 29 design features shown in Table 3.1, we also examined interaction analyses for three potentially moderating variables. First we examined whether gender interacted with any of these features. These analyses were conducted with regression. After statistically controlling for income and negative affect, the main effects of the design characteristic and the moderator variable, respectively, were tested in the model. This was followed by the statistical test for the interaction term (a multiplicative term). So in the case of gender, we regressed housing satisfaction onto the two controls—the specific design characteristic and gender—and then examined the product of the design feature by gender. A significant interaction, net of all of the controls and the two main effects, indicates that the slope of the function between the design characteristic and satisfaction differs according to the level of the moderator variable.

For two of the moderator variables, we found essentially no evidence of salient individual differences. For both men and women, the impacts of all 29 design features were identical. There were no significant interaction terms. It is interesting to note, however, that men were more satisfied, overall, than women were: $F(2, 410) = 9.69$, $p < .001$).

In examining health status, we found one significant interaction. For health status we used the continuous, 10-point magnitude estimation scale from the health ladder (where 1 = very serious health problems and 10 =

in the very best health). For elderly in excellent health (8–10 on the health ladder), the width of interior doorways sufficient for a wheelchair was irrelevant, whereas for those in poor or moderate health, this characteristic was a significant contributor to overall satisfaction with the residence: $F(1, 323) = 8.15, p < .005$. As one might expect, healthier elderly in general were more satisfied with their housing: $F(2, 410) = 3.45, p < .03$.

There were several significant interactions indicating that the impacts of design features on satisfaction varied in relation to the age of the resident. For example, having a fireplace contributed more to the residential satisfaction of the younger elderly (those younger than 70) than it did to that of the moderately old or old old: $F(1, 333) = 4.04, p < .05$.

Similar interaction patterns between age and design characteristic were uncovered for several other design amenities, including having sufficient space for valued possessions: $F(1, 376) = 14.04, p < .001$); having space for personal objects and well-lit displays: $F(1, 374) = 6.45, p < .01$; and having a shower seat: $F(1, 328) = 6.29, p < .01$. In each case the presence of the amenity was tightly tied to satisfaction but only for those who were less than 70 years of age.

On the other hand, two significant interactions revealed the opposite pattern, indicating that the design characteristic was more important for the older-old. For example, good lighting in hallways was strongly related to overall satisfaction only among those older than 70: $F(1,328) = 5.19, p < .02$. For wood trim, satisfaction was unrelated to residential satisfaction for those under 70, but made a difference to others, especially the older elderly, $F(1,332) = 3.82, p < .05$.

IMPLICATIONS FOR THEORY, RESEARCH, AND PRACTICE

Of primary importance in the findings of this study is that housing features significantly contribute to the housing satisfaction of older adults living in the community. Given that finding, what this study contributes to the literature on housing satisfaction is primarily that residential features that address personalization are important elements in housing satisfaction. The two most important independent predictors of housing satisfaction were space for displaying personal possessions and the effective lighting of those displays to ensure they can be seen. These findings suggest that it is not sufficient to examine just housing deficits or the prosthetic capabilities of dwellings. Certainly these features that make a residence livable should be included, but designers also need to consider features that make a residence meaningful and personal. Five of the eight most salient predictors of housing satisfaction were housing features that address meaning. It is also noteworthy that, at least for a sample of relatively healthy elderly people living independently in the community, neither gender nor health status influenced these findings very much. There is some suggestion, however, that with increasing age, some design variables may shift in salience for residential satisfaction. These results should be treated as tentative hypotheses rather than definitive conclusions. We say this for two reasons. First, these analyses are post hoc; they were conducted for exploratory reasons rather than to test specific, a priori hypotheses. Second, a large number of interaction tests yielded only a handful of statistically significant interactions. This raises the possibility of type 1 error, or chance outcome. Clearly, the pattern of the interaction results points to the need for more detailed scrutiny of design variables and satisfaction in relation to age among the elderly.

This study makes several contributions to the literature on housing satisfaction of older adults. In contrast to the larger body of work that focuses on facilities (Francescato, Weidemann, Anderson, & Chenoweth, 1976; Lawton, Nahemow, & Teaff, 1975; Moos and Lemke, 1984; Moos & Lemke, 1994), this study assesses housing satisfaction among older adults living independently in the community. Beyond eliminating the need to generalize facility findings to community dwellings, the fact that housing variability is greater in a community than in facilities enhances the capacity of dwelling features in community-based studies to explain variance in housing satisfaction.

In relation to previous studies of housing satisfaction among community members, the present study expands the spectrum of housing features considered to influence elderly residents' satisfaction with their dwellings. To illustrate, the Perceived Environmental Quality Indices (PEQIs) developed by Christensen and Carp (1987), is composed of highly specific environmental scales. Three scales that emerged as significant predictors of housing satisfaction were the resources for meal preparation scale, the esthetic attributes scale, and the health-related factors scale. Individual items in these scales tended to emphasize function, such as the presence or absence of a four-burner stove and a lighted meter on the cooking top (footcandles). The esthetic resources scale did assess views—the presence or absence of a special or panoramic view from the kitchen—but did not inquire about aesthetic variables such as material and color preferences and display of art work and memorabilia. Jirovec and colleagues (1984) assessed architectural characteristics using a 25-item semantic differential independent-measures instrument. Included were items that spanned a spectrum ranging from aesthetic quality (unique/common) to utility (useful/useless). Architectural characteristics found to be significant predictors of housing satisfaction—preferred texture, modern features, and friendliness—point to the importance of aesthetic factors but do so in such a general way that the findings offer limited design direction. In the present study, both functional and aesthetic features were assessed. Moreover, aesthetic aspects were examined in greater depth than simply asking about pleasing appearance. The issue of aesthetics was linked to personal preferences and expressions of individual identity.

The need remains to transform findings from previous research, the present study, and subsequent work into a heuristic tool that provides useful guidance for practitioners involved in the design of housing in which elderly residents can age in place within the community. A taxonomy for structuring these findings is needed. Ideally, this taxonomy would offer guidance that parallels designers' conceptual thinking during the design process, for concepts are what underlie creative thinking in design. Concepts stimulate creative thought not by tightly defining solutions, but by posing thought-provoking challenges that align with design decisions. The taxonomy presented in this chapter seeks to define conceptual challenges. The structure is a matrix that relates design principles by expanding on a list, authored by Victor Regnier (1994), of the six previously mentioned categories of design decisions that must be made when creating residential interiors for older adults. Ideally, each of these challenges would be addressed first by empirical research that would offer definitive answers. Awaiting that possibility, each challenge can be used to stimulate dialogue between designers and representative elderly residents in the hope that the resulting designs will incorporate the best in conventional wisdom. Table 3.3 conveys the matrix.

CONCLUSION

If the population segment of people older than 65 years of age continues to expand as projected, and if the vast majority of older adults continue to live independently in the community, the residential experience of older community members will be an increasingly important societal issue. Therefore, we need to better understand how specific aspects of the dwellings and their condition contribute to satisfaction with the residential experience of older adults choosing to remain in the community. Moreover, we need better understanding about how satisfaction with the

TABLE 3.3 Design Decisions Matrix

Types of Design Decisions	Spatial Volume and Proportions	Spatial Connections and Circulation	Custom-Built Features	Hardware	Surface Treatments: Materials, Finishes, and Color	Furniture and Equipment	Lighting
Design-Behavior Principles							
Privacy Provide opportunities for regulated social interaction	What ratio of people to rooms supports regulating social interaction?		How can built-in features facilitate regulation of social interaction?				
Social Interaction Provide opportunities for social interaction and communication					How can acoustical properties of materials support communication?	How can furniture arrangement be accommodated so as to support varied social interactions?	

TABLE 3.3 (continued)

Types of Design Decisions	Spatial Volume and Proportions	Spatial Connections and Circulation	Custom-Built Features	Hardware	Surface Treatments: Materials, Finishes, and Color	Furniture and Equipment	Lighting
Choice Promote the resident's control over the environment	How can differentiation of spaces help reinforce choices?			How can design enable varied use to result in differentiated feedback?		How can required forces be matched to varied user strength?	
Safety/Security "Provide an environment that ensures each user will sustain no harm, injury, or undue risk"		How can design of level changes be made to avert accidents?		How can design promote balance?			How can lighting foster safety and reduce risks?
Accessibility and Functioning "Consider manipulation and accessibility as basic requirements for any functional environment"	How can space be minimized yet special mobility needs be accommodated?		How can design of storage acknowledge the physical abilities of the elderly?	How can prosthetic devices help give access and support functioning?			

Adaptability "An adaptable or flexible environment can be made to fit changing personal characteristics"		How can connections be designed to enhance space-use flexibility?	How can built-in storage be designed to make rooms adaptable to different uses?		
Sensory Aspects "Changes in visual, auditory, and olfactory senses should be accounted for in the environment"				How can surface treatments respond to age-related changes in hearing?	How can lighting respond to age-related changes in vision?
Stimulation/Challenge Offer a gradient of stimulation that is challenging and coherent	How can places be created for vicarious experiences?			How can surface treatments be used to create appropriate levels of visual stimulation?	

TABLE 3.3 (continued)

Types of Design Decisions	Spatial Volume and Proportions	Spatial Connections and Circulation	Custom-Built Features	Hardware	Surface Treatments: Materials, Finishes, and Color	Furniture and Equipment	Lighting
Aesthetics/Appearance "Design environments that appear attractive, provoking, and noninstitutional"				How can prosthetic devices be designed not to announce frailty?	How can material types, e.g., wood, be used to foster hominess?		
Legibility/Orientation/Affordances Provide clarity of functional meaning of objects and spaces, and define spatial orientation	How can use of historical reference and local tradition enable design that is familiar and enhances continuity?		How can culturally appropriate custom features foster familiarity?	How can design be made to express intended use?			

Identity Design environments that are personally meaningful and maintain the resident's sense of self	How can space be designed to celebrate valued possessions, e.g., furniture, artwork, and small objects?			How can lighting be designed to illuminate possessions displayed on walls and shelves?
Restoration Provide spaces that support recovery, peace, and serenity		How can visual or physical access to nature be provided?	How can places for contemplation be created?	

residential experience contributes to the psychological well-being of older adults, an interrelationship that research has shown to be important (Evans et al., 2002).

The taxonomy provided in the conclusion of this chapter is intended as a tool for transforming existing and future research into valuable decision-making guidance for practitioners involved in the remodeling or new construction of community-based dwelling units for older adults. Greater insights into critical design issues may also augment elderly residents' decision-making with respect to residential choice or renovations. This study has attempted to contribute to such understanding by expanding the spectrum of housing features considered to be predictors of housing satisfaction. This investigation moves beyond the issue of housing deficits by pointing to the importance not only of features that are functional in nature but also to those that involve personal meaning and reinforce the identity of each resident.

REFERENCES

Altman, I. (1975). *Environment and social behavior*. Monterey, CA: Brocks-Cole.

Bell, A. P., Fisher, J. D., Baum, A., & Greene, T. C. (1996). *Environmental Psychology*. New York: Harcourt Brace College.

Bronfenbrenner Life Course Center, Cornell University. (2000). *Pathways to Life Quality 2000 Combined Data File Codebook*. Ithaca, NY: Cornell University.

Bronfenbrenner Life Course Center, Cornell University. (2000). *Pathways Sample and Variable Descriptions, 2000*. Ithaca, NY: Cornell Unversity.

Butterfield, D., & Weidemann, S. (1987). Housing satisfaction of the elderly. In V. Regnier & J. Pynoos (Eds.). *Housing the aged*. New York: Elsevier.

Carp, F. M., & Christensen, D. L. (1986). Technical environmental assessment predictors of residential satisfaction: A study of elderly women living alone. *Research on Aging, 8*(2), 269–287.

Carp, F. M. (1987). Environment and aging. In D. Stokols & I. Altman (Eds.), *Handbook of environmental psychology*, (Vol. 1, pp. 329–360). New York: Wiley.

Christensen, D. L., & Carp, F. M. (1987). PEQI-based environmental predictors of the residential satisfaction of older women. *Journal of Environmental Psychology, 7*, 45–64.

Christensen, D., Carp. F., Cranze, G., & Wiley, J. (1992). Objective housing indicators as predictors of the subjective evaluations of elderly residents. *Journal of Environmental Psychology, 12*, 225–236.

Eshelman, P., & Evans, G. W. (2002). Home again: Environmental predictors of place attachment and self-esteem for new retirement community residents. *Journal of Interior Design, 28*(1), 1–9.

Evans, G. W., Kantrowitz, E., & Eshelman, P. (2002). Housing quality and psychological well being among the elderly. *Journals of Gerontology*: Pschological Sciences, 57 B(4), P381–383.

Evans, G. W., & McCoy, J. (1998). When buildings don't work: The role of architecture in human health. *Journal of Environmental Psychology, 18*, 85–94.

Francescato, G., Weidemann, S., Anderson, J., & Chenoweth, R. (1976). *Residents' satisfaction in HUD-assisted housing: Design and management factors.* Washington, DC: U.S. Department of Housing and Urban Development.

Golant, S. M. (1982). Individual differences underlying the dwelling satisfaction of the elderly. *Journal of Social Issues, 38*, 121–133.

Jirovec, R., Jirovec, M. M., & Bosse, R. (1984). Architectural predictors of housing satisfaction among urban elderly men. *Journal of Housing for the elderly, 2*(1), 21–32.

Kelly, L. (1955). Consistency of the adult personality. *American Psychologist, 10*, 659.

Lawton, M. P. (1980a). *Environment and aging*. Belmont, CA; Wadsworth.

Lawton, M. P. (1980b). Housing the elderly. *Research on Aging, 2*, 309–328.

Lawton, M. P., Nahemow, L. (1979) Social science methods for evaluating the quality of housing for the elderly. *Journal of Architectural Research, 7*(1), 5–11.

Lawton, M. P., Nahemow, L., & Teaff, J. (1975). Housing characteristic and the well-being of elderly tenants in federally assisted housing. *Journal of Gerontology, 30*(5), 601–607.

Maslow, A. H. (1962). Towards a psychology of being. New York: Harper.

Moos, R. H., & Lemke, S. (1984). Supportive residential settings for older people. In I. Altman, M. P. Lawton, & J. F. Wohlwill (Eds.), *Elderly people and the environment*, (Vol. 7, pp. 159–190). New York: Plenum.

Moos, R. H., & Lemke, S. (1994). Group residences for older adults. New York: Oxford University Press.

Moos, R. H., Lemke, S., & David, T. G. (1987). Priorities for design and management in residential settings for the elderly. In V. Regnier, J. Pynoos (Eds.), *Housing the aged: Design directions and policy considerations* (pp. 179–205). New York: Elsevier.

O'Bryant, S. L., & Wolf, S. M. (1983). Explanation of housing satisfaction of older homeowners and renters. *Research on Aging, 5*, 217–233.

Regnier, V. (1994). *Assisted living housing for the elderly*. New York: Van Nostrand Reinhold.

Struyk, R. J. (1977). The housing situation of elderly Americans. *The Gerontologist, 7*(2), 130–139.

Struyk, R. J., & Turner, M. A. (1984). Changes in the housing situation of the elderly: 1974–1970. *Journal of Housing for the Elderly, 2*(1), 3–19.

Teaff, J. D., Lawton, M. P., Nahemow, L., & Carlson, D. (1978). Impact of age integration on the well-being of elderly tenants in public housing. *Journal of Gerontology, 33*, 126–133.

Toseland, R., & Rasch, J. (1978). Factors contributing to older persons' satisfaction with their communities. *The Gerontologist, 18*, 395–402.

U.S. Bureau of the Census. (1990). *Census of Population and Housing, Special Tabulation on Aging* (STP 14, Tables P52, P57, P59, P61, P63). Washington, DC: U.S.G.P.O.

Vanhorenbeck, S. (1982). *Housing programs affecting the elderly.* Washington, DC: U.S. Government Printing Office.

Watson, D., & Pennebaker, J. W. (1989). Health complaints, stress and distress: Exploring the central role of negative affectivity. *Psychological Review, 96*(2), 234–254.

Weicher, J. C. (1986). Simple measures of inadequate housing. *Journal of Economic and Social Measurement, 14*, 175–195.

Wells, N. M., & Evans, G. W. (1996). Home injuries of people over 65: Risk perceptions of the elderly and those who design for them. *Journal of Environmental Psychology, 16*, 247–257.

Zavotka, S., & Teaford, M. (1997). The design of shared social spaces in assisted living residences for older adults. *Journal of Interior Design, 23*(2), 2–16.

Zhu, L., & Shelton, G. G. (1996). The relationship of housing costs and quality to housing satisfaction of older American homeowners: Regional and racial differences. *Housing and Society, 23*(2), 15–35.

SECTION 3

Role Identities and Social Participation

CHAPTER 4

Roles, Identities, and Residence: Continuity and Changes in Later Adulthood

Phyllis Moen, Donna Dempster-McClain,
Mary Ann Erickson, and Alice Boyce

Both life course and identity theories suggest that life transitions commonly bring changes in roles and, consequently, changes in self-concept (Elder, 1995; Moen, 1995; Mutran & Reitzes 1984). One common transition in later life is residential relocation. While the geographic distribution and migration of older people have been well documented by Longino (2001) and his colleagues (Litwak & Longino, 1987), less information is available about the relationship among the various types of relocation and changes in roles and self-concept.

Litwak and Longino (1987) present a model for interstate migration that focuses on three basic types of moves: amenity moves, which occur during early postretirement years; health-related moves, which occur when moderate forms of disability are experienced; and institutional moves, which take place when health problems overwhelm individuals and their families. The first two types of moves usually find older people leaving their independent family homes in age-integrated neighborhoods and moving to some form of congregate supportive housing, such as planned retirement communities, continuing care retirement communities (CCRCs), adult homes, or one of various types of assisted living facilities (Folts & Streib, 1994; Longino, 2001). Older adults who desire to remain in age-integrated neighborhoods also make moves. These moves can be within or across neighborhoods and are motivated by a variety of wishes, such as to acquire a smaller, more manageable home, apartment, or condo, to move to a more convenient location, or to move closer to adult children.

Documenting the frequency and magnitude of moves among the over-60 population is difficult. According to data from Asset and Health Dynamics, a national survey of older Americans, only about 1 in 20 (5%) moves in any single year, whereas almost 2 in 5 Americans (39%) change residences at some point after age 60 (Schafer, 2000). Pynoos and Golant (1996) estimated that while only about 8% of older people currently reside in planned retirement communities, the number of these communities will continue to increase in the next decade. Also growing is the number of assisted-living facilities in the United States (Sikorska, 1999). Shifts in longevity and lifestyle preferences, along with the aging of the large baby boom cohort, suggest that large numbers of older Americans will be making at least one and perhaps several moves.

Some moves (such as to nursing homes) may be involuntary, whereas moves to retirement communities, CCRCs, or other forms of senior housing, or otherwise downsizing one's independent-living arrangements by moving to a smaller home, are typically voluntary. Nevertheless, even such voluntary relocations produce changes in people's social environments. Older adults moving to congregate housing typically sell the homes in which they raised their children, with some moving away from friends and familiar neighborhoods. In addition, later adulthood moves often entail selling or giving away many possessions as people downsize and move into smaller single-family homes, apartments, condos, or congregate housing. Other important adjustments include the social and psychological as well as the physical changes that take place if the residential transition involves moving from living independently in age-integrated neighborhoods to age-segregated supportive housing (Moen & Erickson, 2001).

We propose that such later-life residential shifts may well affect both the roles people occupy (behavior) and their identities (self-conceptions). There has been little study of the links between being in a role (for example, working for pay) and identifying oneself with a role (such as worker) long after exiting from it (such as through retirement). In fact, the term *identity* is sometimes used to mean *role occupancy*, as if they were one and the same (e.g., Thoits, 1983). But they are not synonymous. Some older people may still see themselves in ways that relate more to their past rather than to their present circumstances. Residential moves may precipitate an abrupt shift in identities as well as in actual role enactments.

In this chapter we use panel data to examine changes in various roles and identities of 682 older adults over a 2-year period (1998–2000). We are interested in the continuity and change in role occupancy (such as being a wife, a volunteer) and identity (seeing oneself as a wife, a volunteer) over time, as well as in the links between identities, role occupancies, and residential circumstances. We consider both where people live and the timing of any recent or earlier housing transition by comparing four groups: (a) stayers, those living in the same (independent) neighborhood housing at both wave 1 and wave 2 of the survey; (b) prior movers to senior housing, those who moved to congregate senior housing facilities prior to wave 1 of the survey and continue to live there throughout the 2-year period between waves; (c) prior movers to a CCRC, those who moved to a CCRC prior to wave 1 or during the 2-year period; and (d) recent movers, those who moved from their neighborhood homes during the 2-year period (between wave 1 and wave 2).

We develop hypotheses based on a life course formulation (which suggests that identities may well reflect an accumulation of experience, including past as well as current roles) in tandem with identity theory (which suggests that identities reflect role salience as indicated by current role occupancy and domains of life satisfaction). Data from the *Pathways to Life Quality* study permits us to investigate the aging self (identity) in the context of both the actual roles people occupy and their residential continuity or change.

THEORY AND HYPOTHESES

Scholars conceptualize identity in terms of both personality traits (usually self-descriptions of traits or typical behaviors) and social roles (based on perceived social locations) (Biddle, 1986; Ferraro, 2001; Turner, 1978). We focus in this chapter on identity in terms of social roles, distinguishing between actual role occupancy (e.g., being a volunteer) and identity (e.g., viewing oneself as a volunteer).

The view of the self as being composed of a number of identities has a long history, beginning with William James (1890). Early role theory emphasized congruence between the self and the social environment, with roles reflecting people's positions in the social structure (Linton, 1936; Parsons, 1951). By contrast, identity theory focuses not on actual roles occupied, but rather on "internalized positional designations" (Stryker 1980, p. 60). Such cognitive identities are organized into a hierarchy of salience. This helps to explain choices among different lines of action including, for example, becoming or remaining a volunteer. The salience of an identity is key to its invocation in any particular situation (Wells & Stryker, 1988). This can also work in reverse. Thus, for example, people who actually engaged in volunteer work are more likely to conceive of themselves as volunteers (Bem, 1970).

A good deal of the identity research of the 1980s and 1990s focused on the structure of social and personal identity. Rosenberg and Gara (1985) proposed a pyramid-shaped model of identities organized by salience, or an individual's commitment to a particular activity associated with an identity. Ogilvie (1987) elaborated upon Rosenberg and Gara's model by investigating the amount of time spent in activities related to major identities and satisfaction with identities in 32 men and women between the ages of 53 and 71. He concluded that the more time spent actually enacting major identities (such as actively volunteering), the higher the level of satisfaction. Deaux (1993) and Reid and Deaux (1996) continue this line of research, focusing on the structure of identity and finding that for college students' social identities (social categories in which individuals claim membership) and personal identities (traits and behaviors that the person finds self-descriptive) are segregated into two distinct categories rather than being integrated. Recently Freund and Smith (1999) investigated spontaneous self-definitions provided by a sample of 516 people, ranging in age from 70 to 103 in the Berlin Aging Study. They found that, regardless of age, the people they interviewed tended to see themselves as being active and present-oriented. Topics raised by these respondents centered around the central themes of life-review, health, and families. Positive emotional well-being was associated with naming more and richer self-defining themes. Whereas these researchers investigated both personality traits and social roles, we focus exclusively on links to actual roles occupied and on residential circumstances to see whether and how they relate to internalized identities.

A life course perspective emphasizes the importance of continuity and change accompanying aging (Elder, 1995; Moen, 2001). In particular, a life course role context approach, (e.g., Herzog, Markus, Franks, & Homberg 1998; Kim & Moen, 2002; Moen, Dempster-McClain, & Williams, 1989, 1992), points to the importance of the social environment in shaping opportunities, expectations, behaviors and self-conceptions. For example, both role continuity and role change (such as remaining or becoming a volunteer) affect people's lifestyle and life quality (Kim & Moen, 2002; Pillemer, Moen, Wethington, & Glasgow, 2000). Residential relocation, as an important later life transition, is often precipitated by changes in physical mobility and health (Longino, 2001; Longino, Jackson, & Zimmerman, 1991; Maddox, 2001).

Residential moves in later life may well be accompanied by psychological and social selection processes (Baltes & Carstensen, 1996; Carstensen, 1992; Rowe & Kahn, 1998) that result in a downsizing not only of place of residence, but also of actual roles and self-conceptions. We propose that later-adulthood residential arrangements, as well as changes in them, matter in terms of the roles people occupy and the identities tied to them. Changes in context often require individuals to actively forge new links between important roles and identities and their new environments (Deaux, 1993). A life course approach suggests that stable living arrangements can lead to stability or even acquisition of identities. Thus people moving to congregate residential environments may experience changes in both role occupancy and identity, but over a period of years may well come to stabilize both the roles they occupy and their sense of self. Accordingly, we propose the following hypotheses:

- Hypothesis 1: Moving within the past 2 years, regardless of type of housing before or after the move, produces an overall reduction in both the number of roles occupied and the number of identities selected.
- Hypothesis 2: Regardless of housing arrangement or moving history, being satisfied with and continuously occupying a particular role increase the likelihood of identifying with that role.
- Hypothesis 3: Prior movers who have lived in senior housing or a CCRC for more than 2 years will maintain or even increase the number of selected identities, especially if they remain in good health.
- Hypothesis 4: Individuals who remain in independent housing (stayers) tend to have stable identities, especially if they remain in good health.

It is to be noted that for the last two hypotheses, we expect health to moderate the relationship between residential status and selected identities.

In previous research on 92 older adults in the *Pathways to Life Quality* study who moved to a CCRC (Moen, Erickson, & Dempster-McClain, 2000), we found role-specific variations in the role behavior and identity relationship. For example, people who were active as volunteers and were satisfied with their volunteer role tended to identify themselves as volunteers. Seeing oneself as a church or synagogue member was associated with regularly attending a church or synagogue. By contrast, seeing oneself as a friend was not related either to role occupancy (being active as a friend) or to satisfaction. In this chapter we build on this previous work in two ways. First, we investigate a larger, more diverse sample, and second, we follow this sample over time, which allows us to examine continuity and change in identities for older adults as they enter and leave particular roles and as they experience both residential continuity and change.

METHODS

SAMPLE

We draw on data from the *Pathways to Life Quality Panel Study* (1998–2000), which looked at individuals ages 56 to 101 in an upstate New York county living in a range of settings, as well as at those who made residential shifts over the past 2 years. The majority of the sample, 57% ($n = 391$), are stayers, having resided continuously and independently in their homes in the same neighborhoods during both waves of the study. Stayers have had a great deal of residential stability throughout their life courses; on average, they have lived in their homes for 27 years (ranging from 2 to 75 years).

Of the sample, 17% ($n = 113$) are prior movers, having lived in senior housing facilities for a minimum of 2 years. In fact, prior movers have lived in congregate residential facilities for an average of 8 years, with a range in years in residence from 2 to 27. Prior movers to a CCRC make up 18% of the sample ($n = 125$). Given that the CCRC in the county studied opened its doors in December of 1995, the length of residency ranges from 2 to 6 years, with an average of 4 years. The majority of the people in this group are founders, those who planned the facility and moved in as soon as it opened.

Recent movers are the smallest group, making up only 8% ($n = 53$) of the sample, averaging only 1.2 years in residence, with a range of 0 to 2 years. Of this group, 32 (60% of the recent movers) moved into a new retirement community consisting of independent apartments in a recently constructed complex with some meals and personal assistance provided, as well as the option, if needed, of moving into an assisted-living section of the facility. Only four (8%) of the recent movers moved into one of seven rural facilities classified as adult homes. Nine (17%) moved within the community, staying in independent homes but changing neighborhoods. Only three of the recent movers moved to another county in New York, with five (9%) moving out of the state. Clearly the recent movers are a diverse group. In some analyses we subdivide recent movers into two groups: those moving to some form of senior housing ($n = 36$) and those moving to other independent-living arrangements ($n = 17$).

MEASURES

In addition to our fourfold categorization of residential dynamics (stayers, prior movers to senior housing, prior movers to a CCRC, and recent movers), we include measures of health, role occupancy, and role identities. We measure perceived health status using the general question "With 10 being very best health and 0 being very serious health problems, which step on the ladder indicates how your health has been lately?" asked in both wave 1 and wave 2.

One section of the interview schedule inquires about current identities. Respondents in wave 1 and wave 2 were given a list of identities and the following instructions: "Here is a list of role identities that are important to individuals at different stages in their lives. Please put an X next to the current role identities that are most important to you at this point in your life." In the strictest sense, we may be capturing identity salience (most important identities) but, as Wells and Stryker (1988) point out, salience itself is a gauge of self-concept.

We investigate both roles (behaviors) and identities (cognitions) in terms of the following: parent, spouse, student, worker, friend, church/synagogue member, grandparent, and volunteer. Questions about current role behaviors for each of these categories are also asked. Occupying the role of spouse is determined by current marital status. Occupying the role of volunteer reflects involvement in volunteer work in the community or residence. Occupying the role of worker reflects working for pay. Occupying the role of student reflects participating in adult education courses. Respondents who attend religious services were coded as occupying a religious role. The last three roles (friend, parent, and grandparent) are based on enacting the role as measured by seeing friends, children, or grandchildren at least weekly. This decision was based on the fact that these roles are less formally institutionalized, and are therefore embodied in the frequency of behavior. To capture continuity and change in role occupancy during the 2-year period between survey waves, we constructed a variable with four categories:

1. moving into or gaining a role;
2. leaving role by wave 2;
3. not in role at either wave 1 or wave 2; and
4. remaining in role at both interview dates.

Similarly, we construct the same four categories for continuity and change of identities. As measures of role quality, we draw on information about respondents' degree of satisfaction with some roles.

ANALYTIC STRATEGY

First we focus on understanding the links between occupying particular roles and identifying with them (that is, rating them as important). Then we narrow our focus to three roles and identities related to a sense of social connectedness within one's community (volunteer, friend, and church/synagogue member) using logistic regression to estimate continuity and change over a 2-year period in these three identities. Our model incorporates both residential and role continuity and change, along with demographic characteristics, health, and role quality. We also investigate possible interaction effects by residential/moving circumstance and health.

RESULTS

DEMOGRAPHIC AND HEALTH CHARACTERISTICS

As shown in Table 4.1, the differences in demographic and health characteristics for the four residential groups are striking. (All differences described are statistically significant at $p < .01$. When important, differences between the two groups of recent movers are mentioned, but data are not shown.) Those who moved recently and the prior movers to a CCRC are the oldest (80.4 years and 79.9 years, respectively), while those who are residentially stable, living independently in the community (stayers) are the youngest (74.0 years). Prior movers living in the CCRC are extremely well educated; more than half (58%) have a graduate degree. In keeping with national trends, the majority of the respondents in each of the groups are women—85% of prior movers to senior housing and 61% of the community stayers. Most (92%) of the prior movers to senior housing live alone, as do more than half (57%) of the recent movers, 2 in 5 (42%) of the prior movers to the CCRC, and 3 in 10 (30%) of those who remain in their independent neighborhood housing. More than 9 in 10 (90%) of the people who moved to senior housing facilities prior to wave 1 (prior movers) are not married, and more than 6 in 10 are widowed. Almost half (48%) of the recent movers to senior housing are also widowed. Income varies in the expected direction, with the CCRC residents having the highest income. Not surprisingly, the community stayers have the highest levels of self-

TABLE 4.1 Demographic, Health, and Role Characteristics by Residential Group

Variable	Stayers (independent neighborhood housing)	Prior movers (senior housing facilities)	Prior movers (continuing care retirement community)	Recent movers	Total sample	Significance
	$n = 391$	$n = 113$	$n = 125$	$n = 53$	$n =$	
Age in 2000						
Mean	74.0 (7.4)	78.8 (7.7)	79.9 (6.3)	80.4 (6.9)	76.4 (7.7)	****a
Median	73.3	78.4	80.2	80.4		
Range	56–101	61–95	63–98	63–92	56–101	
Years in residence	26.9 (16.3)	8.1 (5.1)	3.9 (0.7)	1.2 (0.6)	17.5 (16.6)	***
Education						
H.S. or less	24.6%	54.9%	0.8%	18.9%	25.0	***
College	41.3%	38.1%	41.5%	52.8%	41.8	
Graduate School	34.1%	7.1%	57.7%	28.3%	33.2	
Gender						
Female	60.9%	85.0%	62.4%	71.7%	66.1	***
Male	39.1%	15.0%	37.6%	28.3%	33.9	
Race						
White	98.5%	94.6%	100.0%	98.1%	98.1	***
African-American	1.0%	3.6%	0.0%	1.2		
Other	0.6%	1.8%	0.0%	1.9%	0.7	
Number of identities						
1998	4.3 (1.6)***	3.7 (1.4)	3.3 (1.7)***	3.9 (1.8)	4.0 (1.6)	
2000	4.6 (1.7)	3.9 (1.5)	4.1 (1.7)	3.9 (1.8)	4.3 (1.7)	
Number of roles occupied						
1998	5.4 (1.3)	4.7 (1.4)	4.6 (1.3)***	5.1 (1.4)**b	5.1 (1.4)	
2000	5.3 (1.3)	4.7 (1.0)	5.1 (1.4)	4.7 (1.5)	5.1 (1.4)	

*** wave 1/wave 2 difference within residence/moving significant at $p < .01$.

**b wave 1/wave 2 difference within residence/moving significant at $p < .05$.

reported health (7.7 on a scale of 0–10) drop out of pep and energy (7.2 on a scale of 0–10) and the lowest number of limitations in daily activities (1.4 on a scale of 0–12).

ROLE OCCUPANCY AND IDENTITY IN 1998 AND 2000 BY RESIDENTIAL GROUP

Table 4.1 also presents summary measures of the roles occupied and the identities held at wave 1 and wave 2 by members of each residential group. Looking first at actual role behavior (as opposed to identities), recent movers occupied fewer roles in 2000 than they had in 1998 ($p = < .05$). Specifically, recent movers engaged in an average of 5.1 roles in 1998 (prior to their relocation), dropping to an average of 4.7 in 2000 (after they had moved). This finding supports our prediction (Hypothesis 1) that moving within the past 2 years produces a reduction in role occupancy.

Comparing identities in 1998 and 2000, we find a significant increase in the number of identities for stayers and prior movers to a CCRC. But unlike role behaviors (and contrary to Hypothesis 1) recent movers and prior movers to senior housing remain stable in the number of identities they report.

ROLE OCCUPANCY—CONTINUITY AND CHANGE BY RESIDENTIAL STATUS AND MOVING HISTORY

Table 4.2 describes the continuity and change in role occupancy across the two waves of the survey (from 1998 to 2000). Over half (52%) of the respondents are married at both points in time. A high percentage consistently occupy other roles also: friend (69%), parent (72%), grandparent (85%), volunteer (47%), religious participant (50%), and neighbor (74%). As with identities, the degree of role change is noteworthy, especially role *gain* over the 2-year period. About 13% report that they increased the frequency of seeing friends, started taking classes (taking on the student role), or increased their religious attendance, and 10% began doing volunteer work, thereby moving into the role of volunteer.

Looking at the differences by residential group we find that, between wave 1 and wave 2, stayers in independent neighborhood housing reported gains in three roles: 14% became students, 12% took on the role of friend (they began seeing at least one friend weekly), and 11% became volunteers.

Significant proportions of prior movers to senior housing also began volunteering (10%) and started seeing friends daily (19%). Similarly, many prior movers to the CCRC also gained roles, with increases in seeing friends

TABLE 4.2 Continuity and Change in Identities and Roles, 1998–2000

Identities

Identity	Gaining identity	Losing identity	Not identifying, 1998 or 2000	Identifying, 1998 and 2000	Significant difference by residential group
Spouse	2.5	4.6	42.3	50.5	$p = .000$
Friend	11.5	11.0	4.3	73.2	$p = .000$
Parent	11.8	11.2	12.9	64.1	$p = .000$
Grandparent	11.9	7.5	18.6	62.0	$p = .001$
Volunteer	15.4	10.7	40.6	33.3	NS $p = .11$
Church/synagogue member	9.9	7.5	44.9	37.8	$p = .01$
Worker	17.9	8.9	61.4	11.8	$p = .000$
Student	14.8	2.7	79.6	3.0	NS $p = .07$

Roles

Roles occupied	Gaining role	Leaving role	Not occupying role in 1998 or 2000	Occupying role in 1998 and 2000	Significant difference by residential group
Spouse	0.1	3.4	44.1	52.3	$p = .000$
Friend	13.2	9.5	8.6	68.6	n.s.
Parent	7.9	5.4	14.9	71.8	n.s.
Grandparent	1.9	0.4	12.4	85.2	n.s.
Volunteer	10.7	11.1	31.4	46.8	$p = .008$
Religious participant	12.4	16.7	21.5	49.5	n.s.
Employee	2.7	7.6	75.2	14.5	$p = .000$
Student	12.9	5.0	74.8	7.2	n.s.

daily (31%), seeing children weekly (11%), volunteering (11%), and becoming a student (19%).

Recent movers report role gains in the form of seeing friends daily (26%), volunteering (15%), and becoming a student (15%). But there are several differences between the two groups of recent movers. First, a greater percentage of recent movers who remained in independent neighborhood housing (53% as compared to 31% of the total group) did not volunteer in 1998 or 2000. Second, 20% of recent movers to senior housing, as compared to 11% of the total group, stopped volunteering in 2000.

There is also considerable role continuity from 1998 to 2000. More than 70% of all respondents remain involved with their grandchildren. Stayers, prior movers to senior housing, and recent movers (specifically, movers who remain in independent neighborhood housing) report continuous involvement with their children (the parent role). Prior movers continue with the role of friend; high levels of involvement (over 70%) with friends are reported by both groups of prior movers. Sixty-one percent of prior movers to a CCRC (as compared to 48 percent of the total group) volunteered in both 1998 and 2000. Two roles are far less common in this age group: only 10% or less report continuous involvement as a student or worker.

IDENTITY—CONTINUITY AND CHANGE ON THE BASIS OF RESIDENTIAL STATUS AND MOVING HISTORY

Table 4.2 also presents continuity and change in identities across the two waves of the survey (from 1998 to 2000). For the whole sample, we show the percentage reporting that they gained or lost particular identities. Equally important are the groups that remain stable at both points in time—those who do not hold particular identities in 1998 or 2000 and those who do see themselves as having a particular identity at both points in time.

More than half of the sample selected the identity of spouse (50%), friend (73%), parent (64%) and grandparent (62%) as being important to them at both points in time. Respondents are least apt to hold identities in 1998 and 2000 as worker (61% do not) and student (80% do not). Also noteworthy is the fact that significant proportions of the sample gained the important identities of worker (18%) and volunteer (15%) over the 2-year period. About 11% of the respondents also report losing or no longer list as important their identity as parent, friend, or volunteer (selecting it at wave 1 but not at wave 2).

Next we look at continuity and change in identities by residential status and moving history. We find significant differences (at the bivariate level) in continuity and change in identities by residential group for all except the identities of student and volunteer (see the last column of Table 4.2 for probabilities). Most of the stayers (62%) and the prior movers to the CCRC (58%) see themselves as a spouse at both wave 1 and wave 2. A smaller percentage (38%) of the recent movers and only 10% of the prior movers to senior housing identify themselves in this way at both points. This is closely related to the objective loss of that role (e.g., divorce or the death of the spouse).

The continuous identification of oneself as friend, parent, and grandparent ranges from about 60% to 85% for the four groups, with one exception: only about half of prior movers to the CCRC continuously see themselves as parents (46%) or grandparents (49%). Respondents are less apt to consistently hold more public identities, such as a volunteer (33%) and church or synagogue member (38%). However, there is a real difference with the identity of volunteer among the two subgroups of recent movers: 28% of those moving to senior housing facilities see themselves as volunteers both before and after their move, whereas only 6% of recent movers in the community do so. One other obvious difference stands out: 17% of the stayers continue to identify themselves as workers, while few (only 4 to 7%) in the other groups see themselves as workers at both points in time.

Although one view of aging and of moving to congregate living is a shedding of prior identities, our study shows that a significant proportion of our sample actually gained new identities over the 2 years between interviews. Prior movers to the CCRC show the greatest gain (21% as compared to 12% on average) in identity as friend from 1998 to 2000. This same group also has higher gains in identity as a church member (13% as compared to 10% on average).

IDENTITIES IN 2000

We now turn to multivariate analysis to examine how residential status and moving history, demographic characteristics, role occupancy and change, role satisfaction, and health are related to holding three key identities: friend, volunteer, and church/synagogue member in 2000. We had predicted that continuously occupying a role, as well as being satisfied with it, increases the likelihood of identifying with it (Hypothesis 2), but that the role occupancy/identity relationships might be conditioned by health and residential status and moving history (Hypotheses 3 and 4). Specifically, we expected that prior movers who live in senior housing or a CCRC would maintain or even increase selected identities and that this relationship would be moderated by good health. On the other hand, stayers in independent housing would tend to have stable identities, especially if they remained in good health.

Logistic regression results that predict identifying oneself as a volunteer at time 2 are shown in Table 4.3. Most important for the volunteer identity is actually occupying the role of volunteer over the 2-year period. Those who served as volunteers in both 1998 and 2000 are 20 times more likely than nonvolunteers to hold the identity of volunteer, supporting our second hypothesis. Next most important is moving into that role—becoming a volunteer in the community between waves. Those who do are eight times more apt to identify themselves as volunteers. But prior role enactment also matters for identity. Note that even those who stop volunteering during the 2 years between surveys are more than twice as likely (2.4) to see themselves as volunteers. Those who saw themselves as volunteers in 1998 are three times as likely to hold this identity in 2000, even net of continuity and change in their actual volunteer participation.

As expected (Hypothesis 2), people who are satisfied with their volunteer experiences are more than five times as likely to see volunteer as an important identity. This, too, is net of continuity and change in actual volunteering and their prior (1998) identities.

Consistent with our hypotheses, we find both perceived health and residential/moving status in combination predict whether or not people see themselves as volunteers. The impact of health on identity differs for prior movers to the CCRC and stayers (data not shown). For prior movers to the CCRC, as rating of health increases, so too does the probability of identifying as a volunteer. By contrast, stayers show greater stability in volunteer identity, regardless of health status. Contrary to our hypothesis, the health status of those who moved previously to senior housing is not related to whether or not they see themselves as volunteers.

Also shown in Table 4.3 are the logistic regression results predicting whether respondents hold the identity of friend in 2000. In contrast to the volunteer identity, the friend identity is not predicted by actual role occupancy. But it must be recalled that we measure occupying the friend role by frequency of contact. This may not capture what people interpret as actually enacting a role. For example, some important friendships may be maintained at long distance or with less frequent contact. However, there appears to be some continuity in this internalized identity; those who saw themselves as friends in 1998 are twice as likely to retain that identity in

TABLE 4.3 Odds Ratios for the Regression of Role Occupancy Change, Satisfaction with Role, Moving Status and Health Changes on Selected Identities, 2000

	Volunteer identity	Friend identity	Church member identity
Demographics			
Married	1.7*		
Education		0.8+	
Female	1.5+		
Age			1.0*
Identity 1998	3.1***	2.2**	7.3***
Role occupancy change			
Both 1998 and 2000 (vs. neither 1998 nor 2000)	20.5***	1.0 n.s.	37.5***
Gained role (vs. neither 1998 nor 2000)	7.7***	0.6+	11.2***
Lost role (vs. neither 1998 nor 2000)	2.4***	0.6 n.s.	6.1**
Satisfaction with:			
Community/Volunteer Activities	5.1**		
Friends		3.3**	
Moving Status			
Prior senior housing (vs. stayers)	0.3 n.s.	1.1 n.s.	0.7 n.s.
Prior CCRC (vs. stayers)	.1 *	0.2+	0.5 n.s.
Movers (vs. stayers)	3.7 n.s.	1.1 n.s.	0.1 n.s.
Health			
1998	0.9 n.s.	1.0 n.s.	0.9 n.s.
2000	0.9 n.s.	1.0 n.s.	1.1 n.s.
Health 2000 * move			
Health 2000 * prior movers to senior housing	1.3+	1.1 n.s.	1.0 n.s.
Health 2000 * prior movers to CCRC	1.3*	1.3*	1.1 n.s.
Health 2000 * recent movers	0.9 n.s.	0.9 n.s.	1.3 n.s.

+ $p < .10$; * $p < .05$; ** $p < .01$; *** $p < .001$.
n.s., not significant.

2000. And those expressing satisfaction with their contacts with friends are three times more likely to incorporate the identity of friend into their self-concept.

Both perceived health and moving status in combination again predict whether people see themselves as friends (data not shown). Stayers remaining in their own neighborhood homes over the two waves of the survey tend to retain the identity of friend, regardless of their health, whereas prior movers to the CCRC show an increased probability of holding the friend identity only as ratings of health increase. By contrast, the health status of those who previously moved to senior housing is not related to their identity as friend.

Actual role participation over the 2-year survey period best predicts people's identity as a church/synagogue member. Specifically, time is the most important predictor. Those who report the same frequency of church service attendance over 2 years are 38 times more likely than nonattendees to hold the church member identity. Next most important is increasing attendance over time. Those who start attending religious services more frequently between the two waves of the survey are 11 times more likely to identify themselves as church members. But prior role occupancy matters as well; those who decrease their church attendance are still six times more likely than nonattendees to see themselves as church members. Prior self-concept matters too; those who saw themselves as church members in 1998 are seven times more likely than those who did not to continue to retain that identity in 2000. Neither health nor residential circumstances—alone or in combination (and unlike the other two public statuses we consider)—predicts people's church member identity.

DISCUSSION AND IMPLICATIONS FOR RESEARCH

Studies of social integration (see, for example, Moen & Fields, 2002; Pillemer, Moen, Wethington, & Glasgow, 2000; Thoits, 1983) point to the importance to people's psychological and perceived identity of both actually occupying roles and of holding particular identities. What is less clear are the links between objective roles and perceived identities over time. In this chapter we have shown they are related, but in complex ways that depend on people's health, residential circumstances, and moving history, as well as on the particular role and identity relationship investigated.

Our goal in this chapter has been to promote understanding of the relationships among these factors—roles, identities, health, and residence—among the respondents in the *Pathways to Life Quality* study. What we find first is considerable fluidity in both the roles and the identities over the 2-year survey period. This suggests that continuity theory might best incorporate a dynamic life course perspective to explain processes of identity development and social ties in later adulthood. One thing is clear: older Americans both retain and gain roles and identities as they age.

Our evidence also points to the importance of viewing roles and identities as different, but related, phenomena. To be sure, staying in or taking on a particular role (such as being a volunteer) is related to holding a particular identity (such as seeing oneself as a volunteer). But even those who let go of a particular role are likely to retain the identity associated with it. Clearly, roles as objective behaviors and identities as internalized locations are *not* identical.

Third, both residential location and residential change matter in conjunction with people's health. Thus we find that stayers in residential neighborhoods show the greatest stability in identity as both volunteer and friend, regardless of their health status. In contrast, for those prior movers living in the CCRC, as their health ratings increase so does the probability that they see themselves as volunteers or friends. Our analyses, like those in other chapters in this volume, also show the heterogeneity of the congregate living experience. Not only do residents of a continuing care community differ, in terms of the roles and identities they hold, from those in other living arrangements, but recent movers to the CCRC differ from longer-term residents in the same facility.

The next steps in research and theory building involve specifying the biographical careers of both role careers and identity careers as each unfolds over time and as they intersect with one another and with concurrent life changes. It is important to recognize that both role change and residential change are dynamic processes. For example, residential location involves several phases—considering whether to move or stay in one's current location, deciding to move, planning the move, actually executing the move, and settling in (Young, 1998).

Knowing about changes and continuities in subjective identities and actual role behaviors tells us little about their interface. For example, do individuals who start volunteering between various waves of data collection also begin to take on the identity of volunteer? Does length of time in a role matter in terms of taking on a particular identity? Longitudinal studies of these issues and their relationships to changes in health as well as to residential and other shifts in people's physical and social environment can illuminate the dynamic involved in the links between physical location (such as residential environment), social location (such as roles enacted), and internalized location (such as subjective identities).

IMPLICATIONS FOR PRACTICE AND POLICY

Our results have important implications for the ways American institutions create and sustain what it means to grow old in contemporary society. First, the people we interviewed in the *Pathways to Life Quality* study gained as well as lost roles and identities, even over as short a period as 2 years. Later years of adulthood are not simply a time of role (or identity) loss, and they should not be viewed as such. Moreover, distinguishing between objective roles and subjective identities is important, given the tendency of professionals and practitioners to view older clients only in terms of current, rather than past, circumstances.

The pragmatic issue is how to sustain and encourage the vital role involvements and identities that research consistently shows to be important for life quality. New social inventions are required, arrangements that tap the potential of the growing numbers of educated, vigorous, and talented people in their 60s, 70s, and 80s, and beyond (Freedman, 2000; Moen, 2003). Community programs such as Offices for the Aging, and programs in congregate facilities are only a very small beginning. New ideas and new arrangements make sense as Americans are living longer and as baby boomers are beginning to move into retirement.

Second, residential changes as well as role changes (such as retirement) may be key points of both vulnerability and opportunity. Thinking of ways to encourage volunteering, friendship formations, and religious involvement may be especially important for people in residential transition. Part of the difficulty that older people experience as they move into new living environments (or leave their primary career jobs) may be the mismatch between their new lifestyles and their (old) identities. Providing opportunities and encouragement to continue participation in and identification with meaningful roles can ease this transition. For example, we find that people living in a CCRC actually tend to increase their participation as friend, volunteer, and student over time.

One problem with focusing on the benefits of social roles is an assumption that "more is better" for every individual. However, research points to the importance of formal integrative roles (such as community participant) that provide opportunities for productive—and social—engagements. Encouraging volunteer community participation is beneficial for all concerned. From a policy standpoint, programs encouraging volunteer community participation are low in cost and can benefit a number of groups. Creating opportunities for older people to tutor at-risk youth, for example, benefits both generations and reduces the burdens on schools.

The helping professionals who want to enrich the lives of older adults but don't want to alienate those who are not interested might use identities as a way of targeting opportunities for social participation. For example, people who hold certain identities such as volunteer but are not actually engaged in volunteering may be easily recruited into community service. But we repeat: small programs cannot change the mindset of a nation that persists in placing older people on the sidelines of society. New institutional arrangements are needed—circumstances that provide people with meaningful roles and identities regardless of age or residential location.

Third, the story that is beginning to emerge is neither simple nor straightforward; nor are any of the solutions proposed for creating or sustaining vital engagement and meaningful identities in later adulthood. In this chapter we have begun to illuminate the complicated links among health, residential shifts, roles, and self-conceptions. Successful aging (e.g., Baltes & Carstensen, 1996; Rowe & Kahn, 1998) is a life-long and dynamic process of change in social location, psychological location, and residential location. But it is also a process embedded in obsolete, age-graded role and identity expectations that no longer fit contemporary reality.

REFERENCES

Baltes, M. M., & Carstensen, L. L. (1996). The Process of Successful Aging. *Aging and Society, 16*, 397–422.

Bem, D. J. (1970). *Beliefs, Attitudes, and Human Affairs*. Belmont, CA: Brooks/Cole.

Carstensen, L. L. (1992). Social and emotional patterns in adulthood: Support for socioemotional selectivity theory. *Psychology and Aging, 7*, 331–338.

Biddle, B. J. (1986). Recent developments in role theory. *Annual Review of Sociology, 12*, 67–92.

Deaux, Kay. (1993). Reconstructing social identity. *Personality and Social Psychology Bulletin, 19*, 4–12.

Elder, G. H., Jr. (1995). The life course paradigm: Social change and individual development. In P. Moen, G. H. Elder, Jr., & K. Luscher (Eds.), *Examining lives in context: Perspectives on the ecology of human development*, (pp. 101–139). Washington, DC: American Psychological Association.

Ferraro, K. F. (2001). Aging and role transitions. In R. H. Binstock & L. K. George (Eds.), *Handbook of Aging and the Social Sciences* (pp. 313–330). San Diego: Academic.

Folts, W. E., & G. F. Streib. (1994). Leisure-oriented retirement communities. In W. E. Folts & D. E. Yeatts (Eds.), *Housing and the aging population: Options for the new century* (pp. 121–144). New York: Garland.

Freedman, M. (1999). *Prime time: How baby boomers will revolutionize retirement and transform America.* New York: Public Affairs.

Freund, A. M., & Smith, J. (1999). Content and function of the self-definition in old and very old age. *Journal of Gerontology, 54B,* P55–P67.

Herzog, A. R., Markus, H. R., Franks, M. M., & Homberg, D. (1998). Activities and well-being in older age: Effects of self-concept and educational attainment. *Psychology and Aging, 13*(2), 179–185.

James, W. (1890). *The principles of psychology.* New York: Holt.

Kim, J., & Moen, P. (2002). Retirement transitions, gender, and psychological well-being: A life-course, ecological model. *Journal of Gerontology: Psychological Sciences, 57B,* P212–P222.

Linton, R. (1936). *Study of man.* New York: Appleton-Century.

Litwak, E., & Longino, C. F., Jr. (1987). Migration patterns among the elderly: A developmental perspective. *The Gerontologist, 27,* 266–272.

Longino, Charles F. Jr. 2001. Geographical distribution and migration. In R. H. Binstock & L. K. George (Eds.), *Handbook of aging and the social sciences* (pp. 103–124). San Diego: Academic.

Longino, C. F., Jr., Jackson, D., & Zimmerman, R. (1991). The second move: Health and geographic mobility. *Journals of Gerontology, 46S,* 218–224.

Maddox, G. L. (2001). Housing and living arrangements: A transactional perspective. In R. H. Binstock & L. K. George (Eds.), *Handbook of aging and the social sciences* (pp. 426–443). San Diego: Academic.

Moen, P. (1995). A life course approach to post-retirement roles and well-being. In L. A. Bond, S. J. Cutler, & A. E. Grams (Eds.), *Promoting successful and productive aging* (pp. 239–256). Thousand Oaks, CA: Sage.

Moen, P. (2001). The gendered life course. In R. H. Binstock & L. K. George (Eds.), *Handbook of Aging and the Social Sciences* (5th ed., pp. 179–196). San Diego, CA: Academic.

Moen, P. (2003). Midcourse: Navigating retirement and a new life stage. In J. Mortimer & M. J. Shanahan (Eds.), *Handbook of the life course.* New York: Plenum.

Moen, P., Dempster-McClain, D., & Williams, R. M. Jr. (1989). Social integration and longevity: An event history analysis of women's roles and resilience. *American Sociological Review, 54,* 635–647.

Moen, P., Dempster-McClain, D., & Williams, R. M. Jr. (1992). Successful aging: A life course perspective on women's multiple roles and health. *American Journal of Sociology, 97,* 1612–1638.

Moen, P., & Erickson, M. A. (2001). Decision-making and satisfaction with a continuing care retirement community. *Journal of Housing for the Elderly, 14,* 53–69.

Moen, P., Erickson, M. A., & Dempster-McClain, D. (2000). Social role identities among older adults in a continuing care retirement community. *Research on Aging, 22*(5), 559–579.

Moen, P., & Fields, V. (2002). Midcourse in the United States: Does unpaid community participation replace paid work? *Ageing International, 27*, 21–48.

Mutran, E., & Reitzes, D. C. (1984). Intergenerational support activities and well-being among the elderly: A convergence of exchange and symbolic interaction perspectives. *American Sociological Review, 49*, 117–130.

Ogilvie, D. M. (1987). Life satisfaction and identity structure in late middle-aged men and women. *Psychology and Aging, 2*, 217–224.

Parsons, T. (1951). *The Social System*. New York: Free.

Pillemer, K., Moen, P., Wethington, E., & Glasgow, N. (Eds.). (2000). *Social Integration in the Second Half of Life*. Baltimore: Johns Hopkins University.

Pynoos, J., & Golant, S. (1996). Housing and living arrangements for the elderly. In R. Binstock & L. George (Eds.), *Handbook of aging and the social sciences* (pp. 303–324). San Diego, CA: Academic.

Reid, A., & Deaux, K. (1996). Relationship between social and personal identities: Segregation or integration? *Journal of Personality and Social Psychology, 71*, 1084–1091.

Rosenberg, S., & Gara, M. A. (1985). The multiplicity of personal identity. In P. Shaver (Ed.), *Review of personality and social psychology* (Vol. 6, pp. 87–113). Beverly Hills, CA: Sage.

Rowe, J. W., & Kahn, R. L. (1998). *Successful aging*. New York: Random House.

Schafer, R. (2000). *Housing America's seniors*. Cambridge, MA: Joint Center for Housing Studies of Harvard University.

Sikorska, E. (1999). Organizational determinants of resident satisfaction with assisted living. *The Gerontologist, 39*(4), 450–456.

Stryker, S. (1980). *Symbolic interactionism: A social structural version*. Menlo Park, CA: Benjamin/Cummings.

Thoits, P. A. (1983). Multiple identities and psychological well-being: A reformulation and test of the social isolation hypothesis. *American Sociological Review, 48*, 174–187.

Turner, R. H. (1978). The role and the person. *American Journal of Sociology, 84*, 1–23.

Wells, L. E., & Stryker, S. (1988). Stability and Change in Self Over the Life Course. In P. Baltes, D. Featherman, & Lerner (Eds.), *Life span development and behavior* (pp. 191–229). Hillsdale, NJ: Erlbaum.

Young, H. (1998). Moving to congregate housing: The last chosen home. *Journal of Aging Studies, 12*(2), 149–165.

CHAPTER 5

Social Participation and Integration

Mary Ann Erickson and Phyllis Moen

The social integration of individuals into the larger society—or, conversely, their social isolation from it—has long been a topic of social research. Recognizing what Rosow (1967) termed the "roleless role" of life after retirement, gerontologists have focused on the perceived and actual social integration of older individuals, a group particularly at risk for isolation (see reviews in Pillemer, Moen, Wethington, Glasgow, 2000). A number of studies have linked social integration (in terms of multiple role involvements or the enactment of particular roles such as formal volunteering) with longevity, good health, and psychological well-being (e.g., Herzog, House, & Morgan, 1991; Moen, 1995; Moen, Dempster-McClain, & Williams, 1989, 1992; Musick, Herzog, & House, 1999). This evidence underscores the importance of actual role participation for the health and well-being of those in their later adult years. Moreover, a sense of connectedness (perceived integration) has also been related to psychological well-being (e.g., Liang, Dvorkin, Kahana, & Mazian, 1980; Mancini & Blieszner, 1992).

We in the United States confront two conflicting dynamics. Major trends in educational attainment, health, and longevity as well as increasingly early retirement mean that those in their 60s, 70s, and 80s are better educated, healthier, more vital, and "younger" than ever before. On the other hand, Americans who have retired from their primary career jobs are at risk of being pushed out of the mainstream of society. This reflects the structural lag in the provision of meaningful role involvements for Americans in the later years of adulthood. (For a discussion of structural lag, see Riley & Riley, 1994.) Older Americans on the whole may be more able to contribute to the broader society than was true of their parents or their grandparents but, like their parents and grandparents, are more apt to be on the sidelines of society, unable to participate in paid or unpaid forms of productive engagement in any formal, sustained, or meaningful way (Young & Glasgow, 1998).

Increasing heterogeneity in where older Americans live may affect both their inclination and their opportunities for role participation. Most older people are living in the same age-diverse neighborhoods as they did in midlife, but growing numbers are moving to various forms of congregate housing (Folts & Yeatts, 1995; Moen & Erickson, 2001). Whether or not people in differing living arrangements are equally likely to be *objectively* socially integrated (in terms of actual role enactments) or to feel *subjectively* connected to others is an issue we address in this chapter. Living arrangements, and particularly changing living arrangements, may also affect older people's ability to maintain these different kinds of connections over time. To examine variations in social integration on the basis of residential arrangement we draw on two resources: a panel study of older adults (ages 70–100) living both in the larger community and in group housing; and theoretical paradigms of the life course and the ecology of human development.

KEY CONCEPTS

Social integration is a concept historically applied to collectivities (Williams, 1965), but it is one that can also describe the multiple roles of individuals. A distinction can be made between social-psychological integration and structural integration, with structural integration connoting the concrete role involvements of individuals. Psychological integration, on the other hand, is the subjective experience of connectedness with one's larger community. Both concepts are related; both may be important in predicting health outcomes.

The behavior enacted in fulfilling a position with defined rights and responsibilities constitutes a role (Linton, 1936; Williams, 1965). Older adults may occupy a range of roles—such as worker, spouse, churchgoer, friend, club member, parent, volunteer, neighbor—each with its own attendant behavioral (role) expectations. Some roles, such as that of worker, are highly structured whereas others, such as friend or neighbor, are diffuse, with more vaguely defined obligations and privileges rather than highly specified rights and duties.

Multiple roles is a concept isomorphic with Merton's (1968) notion of *status set*, referring to the "complex of distinct positions assigned to individuals both within and among social systems" (p. 434). The greater number of roles, by definition, the greater the level of social connectedness or integration. This conforms to House and Kahn's (1985) use of the term *social integration* or, conversely, *isolation*, to represent "the existence or quantity of relationships" (p. 85). Multiple role involvements can be seen as a protective mechanism, like socioeconomic status. This protective mechanism is related, broadly, to a variety of components of health, bolstering a sense of well-being over the life course. Conversely, the absence of role involvements and its accompanying social isolation is a significant risk factor for the development of disease and health impairment. However, it is not clear whether actually occupying particular or multiple roles or simply feeling a subjective sense of integration is more important. This is analogous to the question of whether perceived social support or received social support buffers stressful life events (Wethington & Kessler, 1986).

THEORETICAL FRAMEWORK

The life course and ecology of human development perspectives (e.g., Bronfenbrenner, 1995; Elder, George, & Shanahan, 1996; Moen & Fields, 1999) point not only to the importance of context (such as individual or group living arrangements) but also to the potential for shifts in perceptions and behavior accompanying major life transitions (such as moving to a group living arrangement), and the dynamic nature of roles and relationships. Thus we can consider continuity and change in social integration (both the objective roles and the subjective sense of connectedness) in terms of a "career." Integration changes over time in conjunction with residential circumstances, while residential circumstances change over the life course in conjunction with shifting opportunities, inclinations, and experiences.

The notion of *cumulation of advantage or disadvantage* (e.g., Moen, 2001; Moen et al., 2000; O'Rand, 1996) underscores continuity over the life course, with those older people who are already socially integrated most apt to continue being so. Since scholars have found social integration to be most common among those advantaged in other ways in society, we anticipated that older adults with high levels of education and with few health limitations would be involved in more roles (including paid work and volunteering) and would perceive themselves as being more socially connected than would those with fewer such resources, regardless of their current residential arrangements.

CONTEXTS AND CONTINGENCIES

The life course and ecology of human development orientations point to the heterogeneity of older adults' life paths, how they differ by age and gender, and how they are shaped by life contexts and contingencies, including residential arrangements. Some older Americans are more integrated than others, depending on the opportunities and constraints of their environments as well as on their own motivations and capabilities. The life course perspective also suggests that changes in these environmental contexts can lead to changes in older adults' life paths.

Certain roles can prove advantageous to life quality. For instance, more informal roles involving primary groups, such as the roles of relative, friend, and neighbor, may offer emotional support that is beneficial to psychological well-being (Litwak et al., 1989). Participation in these roles also may serve as a source of information and advice as well as provide more concrete forms of assistance from others (House & Kahn, 1985). Such social bonds have been found to promote mental health (Aneshensel & Frerichs, 1982; Brown & Harris, 1978) and reduce mortality (Berkman & Breslow, 1983; House, Robbins & Metzner, 1982). These findings suggest that roles providing social support, rather than the total number of roles, that are important facilitators of both subjective integration and well-being.

Other research suggests that particular roles in the public sphere, such as employment and community volunteer participation, are more important than simply the aggregate number of roles held by individuals. Employment has been shown to be positively linked to women's mental and physical health (e.g., Gove & Geerken, 1977; Kessler & McRae, 1982; Nathanson, 1980; Verbrugge, 1983, 1985) and may have a greater impact on the subjective sense of connectedness than other roles. However, employment may be less consequential for either subjective integration or well-being once individuals are in their 70s, 80s, and 90s. Similarly, participation in volunteering, especially formal community service through an organization (rather than simply helping out one's neighbor), has been related to psychological health and longevity (e.g., Moen, Dempster-McClain, & Williams, 1989, 1992; Musick, Herzog, & House, 1999).

Other roles may also be salient for the subjective integration of this age group. Older adults who see friends frequently or those who attend church regularly may feel a high degree of social connectedness, regardless of what other roles they may occupy.

Three contexts and contingencies cannot be ignored in linking objective role participation to subjective psychological integration: (a) individual dispositions and resources; (b) family structure, stresses, and supports; and (c) the opportunities, culture, and constraints of various residential arrangements. Other key contextual factors are (d) age and gender. Changes in these factors may precipitate changes in perceived and actual integration, as discussed subsequently.

INDIVIDUAL RESOURCES

Personal resources such as education and health are typically associated with higher levels of social integration (Brown & Harris, 1978). This reflects the social gradient, with those higher up the status ladder advantaged in their life quality. Structural integration, enacting roles, becomes a resource as well, promoting psychological integration. In fact, our model sees structural integration as a key mediator between role occupancy and psychological integration (Figure 5.1). From a more dynamic perspective, changes in health or in roles occupied should produce corresponding gains or losses in the sense of psychological integration.

FAMILY CIRCUMSTANCES

A life course, ecological approach challenges researchers to consider the family context of social integration. Ties with children and the presence of a supportive spouse may well promote both structural and psychological integration. On the other hand, some family responsibilities, such as caregiving for an infirm spouse, may actually dampen both objective and subjective integration. Family circumstances may also be key for psychological integration, whether or not individuals have other role involvements. Becoming widowed may certainly be a crucial event in reducing integration.

RESIDENTIAL CONTEXTS AND THE OPPORTUNITY STRUCTURE

Research suggests that the features of particular living arrangements can foster or constrain the social integration of older adults (Erickson, Dempster-McClain, Whitlow, & Moen, 2000). For example, opportunities for individuals to participate in formal volunteering may well differ depending on

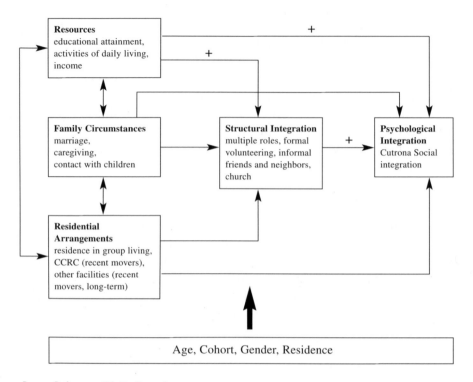

Source: *Pathways to Life Quality* study.

Figure 5.1 Estimating the structural and psychological social integration of older adults in various living arrangements.

the type of residential environment and the recency of the move. Similarly, opportunities for creating and maintaining informal social contacts differ with residential context. Residents of congregate housing are in much closer proximity to others than residents of independent housing in the community. While this proximity does not guarantee a higher level of structural or psychological integration, it may make it easier for many (Lee, Oropesa & Kanan, 1994).

THE SIGNIFICANCE OF AGE AND GENDER

Social systems use both age and gender as fundamental bases for social organization. Despite the push toward gender equality and policies directed against age discrimination, cultural norms persist in defining sex-appropriate behavior and in shaping distinctive age-graded life pathways for women and men (Moen, 2001). It cannot be assumed, therefore, that social integration in terms of multiple roles, or the factors producing a subjective sense of connectedness, are similar for both sexes or for those in their 70s compared to older adults in their 80s and 90s.

Durkheim (1897/1951) observed that women were less involved than men in collective existence and, consequently, less likely to reap either the benefits or the costs of that involvement. The same can be said for the older-old, compared to the younger-old. Moreover, as women age they are increasingly likely to be widowed, so other role involvements (beyond that of spouse) become increasingly significant to their sense of subjective integration.

HYPOTHESES

Figure 5.1 summarizes our theoretical model. We view structural integration as both an outcome of various ecologies and processes and a mediator of psychological integration. We also view age cohort, gender, and residence as key moderators.

To sum up our theoretical argument: the life course and ecology of human development perspectives offer complementary—contextual, dynamic, and developmental—views of possible links between the residential locations of older adults and their social integration. First, location may not be significantly related to social integration; what may matter most for both structural and psychological integration are the resources individuals bring to later adulthood, resources associated with a cumulation of advantage. In fact, residential location itself may simply reflect the choices and opportunities of people with varying amounts of resources. This suggests the following hypotheses:

- Hypothesis 1: Higher educational training and health, including changes in the ability to perform everyday activities, best predict changes in social integration, regardless of residential arrangements, moves, age, or gender.
- Hypothesis 2: Structural integration, in terms of increases or declines in involvement in nonfamily roles as well as the enactment of particular roles (especially paid work and unpaid community participation), predicts changes in psychological integration, mediating any effects of residential arrangement or moves.

A second way of framing the issue is in terms of the stressful transitions, particularly residential change. This approach would lead to the following hypotheses:

- Hypothesis 3: Older adults who recently (within the past 2 years) moved to group housing are the least likely to be structurally or psychologically integrated.
- Hypothesis 4: Older adults residing in their own individual neighborhood homes (typically long-term arrangements) would be the most integrated both structurally and psychologically compared to those in group living arrangements.

These theoretical paradigms also suggest the importance of family, gender, and age contexts and lead to the following hypotheses:

- Hypothesis 5: Marriage should promote the psychological integration of men and women, regardless of their objective role involvements.
- Hypothesis 6: Older women who are not married will feel more psychologically integrated to the degree to which they have objective role involvements.
- Hypothesis 7: Women and men in their 80s and 90s will be less apt either to be structurally integrated or to feel psychologically integrated, compared to those in their 70s, regardless of where they live.

We suggest that these hypotheses help explain continuity and change in integration over time. Higher education, marriage, younger age, and less residential disruption should be associated with maintaining structural and psychological integration over time as well as influencing levels at one point in time.

RESEARCH DESIGN

SAMPLE

To address the factors related to both structural and psychological integration, and the links between the two, we analyze data collected in 1997–98 and 1999–2000 as part of the *Pathways to Life Quality* study. We include only cases that have data for both interviews. We also exclude those living continuously in assisted-living residences and those who moved to nursing homes between interviews, and we truncate the random community sample to those 70 and older.

Because we hypothesize that the recency of a residential move will affect social integration, our groups for analysis reflect years in housing as well as residential location. We eliminated 20 cases of respondents who moved to different housing arrangements between interviews, but kept the group of 37 respondents who moved from the community to the independent/assisted-living complex. The five groups in our analysis are: older community residents (age 70 and older, $n = 226$); long-term residents of senior housing (5 years or more, $n = 66$); shorter term residents of senior housing (2–5 years, $n = 43$); residents of the continuing care retirement community (2–5 years in residence, $n = 125$); and movers to the independent/assisted-living complex (2 years or fewer in residence, $n = 37$).

MEASURES

Structural integration is operationalized both as an aggregate measure and by individual measures. We focus on nonfamily roles only as these are the roles that are generally voluntary and more subject to change over time than are family roles (spouse, parent, grandparent). Our measure of nonfamily roles adds one point for each of the following: employed, club member, volunteer, see friends almost every day, see neighbors almost every day, and attend religious services twice a month or more (see chapter 5). We measure four levels of community participation—formal (those who volunteer and belong to at least one organization); informal (those who volunteer only); member only (no volunteering); and no participation. Individual items are single questions. For frequency of contact with children and relatives, those without children or relatives are coded "never."

We measure psychological integration using the Social Integration subscale of the Social Provisions Scale (Cutrona & Russell, 1987). The four items in the scale are (a) I feel part of a group; (b) There are people who enjoy the same activities I do; (c) No one shares my interests or concerns; and (d) No one likes to do the things I do. Responses are 1, Strongly disagree through 4, Strongly agree. The reliability of this scale (Chronbach's alpha) is .77.

We operationalize functional limitations as the number of everyday tasks that respondents report are limited because of a physical or mental condition. The possible choices are walking six blocks, climbing a flight of stairs, performing day-to-day household tasks, moving about the house and yard, caring for personal needs (such as eating and bathing), going grocery shopping, keeping a doctor's appointment, doing volunteer work, driving a car, doing usual recreational activities, using public transportation, and bending, kneeling, or stooping.

ANALYTIC STRATEGY

We use ordinary least squares regression and logistic regression to examine the relationships between (a) resources, family circumstances, residential context, and age and gender and (b) structural and psychological interaction. We also investigate possible interaction effects in the models.

FINDINGS

STRUCTURAL INTEGRATION

In addition to the demographic differences among residential groups covered in previous chapters, there are differences in the structural integration of respondents in various living environments (Table 5.1). Continuing care retirement community (CCRC) residents tend to have the highest number of nonfamily roles (2.9 in 1998; 3.6 in 2000), followed by long-term residents of senior housing (3.0 in 1998; 3.2 in 2000). Older community residents and movers to the independent/assisted-living complex reported a lower number of nonfamily roles (2.0 in 1998; 2.6 and 2.8 in 2000, respectively), while short-term residents of senior housing were between the extremes. Note that the average number of roles increased in each group, even for those who moved to group housing between interviews. (The format of the questions about how often respondents see friends and neighbors was changed between interviews. In 1998 the responses were categorical, whereas in 2000 the response was an estimate of days per month. This change in format may have contributed to the increase across groups in these variables.) Refer to chapter 4 on role identities.

Focusing on various forms of role involvements, we see residential differences in the role of paid worker. Older community residents and CCRC residents are most likely to be employed. This is true for both age cohorts (70–79 and 80+). In addition, older residents in the community and CCRC residents seemed most likely to maintain their employment over the 2-year study period.

We considered three forms of community participation: formal volunteering (a combination of volunteering with formal organizational membership); informal volunteering (helping out, without any organizational tie); and membership in an organization (such as bridge clubs, with no civic volunteer activity). The CCRC residents are the most likely to participate in formal volunteer activities, with about half (48%) of CCRC respondents doing so. While the distribution across various forms of community participation stayed remarkably stable for the CCRC residents, for-

TABLE 5.1 Structural Integration, Family Roles, and Psychological Integration by Residential Groups, 1998 and 2000

Variable	Older community residents	Long-term senior housing	Short-term senior housing	CCRC residents	Movers to IAL complex	F or Pearson chi-square
Structural integration						
Nonfamily roles 1998	2.0 (1.3)	3.0 (1.4)	2.5 (1.4)	2.9 (1.2)	2.0 (1.2)	13.4***
Nonfamily roles 2000	2.6 (1.4)	3.2 (1.2)	3.0 (1.2)	3.6 (1.2)	2.8 (1.4)	12.1***
Worker (employed) 1998	16.6	9.4	9.3	14.5	5.4	5.5
Worker (employed) 2000	15.0	1.5	4.7	12.0	2.7	14.7**
Community participation 1998				34.9***		
Formal volunteer	27.6	27.7	16.3	48.4	18.9	
Informal volunteer	24.0	30.8	30.2	25.0	37.8	
Org. member only	12.4	6.2	7.0	7.3	10.8	
No participation	36.0	35.4	46.5	19.4	32.4	
Community participation 2000				43.1***		
Formal volunteer	38.9	30.3	30.2	47.6	27.8	
Informal volunteer	9.0	21.2	18.6	25.0	19.4	
Org. member only	21.3	9.1	7.0	8.1	19.4	
No participation	30.8	39.4	44.2	19.4	33.3	
Religious attender (weekly) 1998	51.6	47.7	51.2	40.0	56.8	7.1
Religious attender (weekly) 2000	53.3	50.0	47.6	33.1	48.6	21.2**
Friend (see almost daily) 1998	20.1	66.2	40.5	53.8	18.9	94.8***
Friend (see almost daily) 2000	42.4	75.8	51.2	81.6	41.7	81.2***

TABLE 5.1 (continued)

Variable	Older community residents	Long-term senior housing	Short-term senior housing	CCRC residents	Movers to IAL complex	F or Pearson chi-square
Neighbor (see almost daily) 1998	20.2	81.3	76.7	49.2	27.0	123.0***
Neighbor (see almost daily) 2000	31.1	90.0	93.0	92.8	89.2	198.3***
Family roles						
Percent married 1998	58.0	12.1	16.3	63.2	40.5	72.7***
Percent married 2000	55.3	7.6	14.3	57.6	37.8	71.9***
Contact children (month) 1998	11.8 (11.9)	10.0 (13.2)	12.7 (11.8)	7.8 (8.8)	11.1 (11.1)	3.0*
Contact children (month) 2000	10.4 (11.0)	6.6 (7.8)	7.4 (8.9)	2.7 (3.3)	4.2 (5.4)	17.0***
Relatives almost daily (%) 1998	14.0	12.3	25.6	5.8	13.5	31.6*
Relatives almost daily (%) 2000	17.3	6.1	9.3	8.0	8.1	24.0
Percent caregiving 1998	8.0	9.2	9.3	18.5	2.8	12.4*
Percent caregiving 2000	16.4	15.4	11.9	7.3	13.9	6.0
Psychological integration						
1998	3.2 (0.4)	3.1 (0.4)	3.0 (0.4)	3.3 (0.4)	3.1 (0.5)	3.5**
2000	3.2 (0.4)	3.1 (0.4)	3.0 (0.4)	3.2 (0.4)	3.0 (0.3)	3.9**
n	226	66	43	125	37	

$* p < .05; ** p < .01; *** p < .001.$
CCRC, continuing care retirement community.

mal volunteering tended to be greater in the other residential groups. In most cases it seemed to be that informal volunteers moved into formal volunteering; the percentages of nonparticipants stayed very much the same between interviews for most groups. Shorter term residents of senior housing were the least likely to participate formally or informally in community service or other activities (46.5% in 1998; 44.2% in 2000). These respondents were the most vulnerable to structural isolation in terms of not being engaged in formal volunteering, informal helping out, or social club activities. Least at risk for such social isolation (in terms of occupancy of at least one of these roles) were the residents of the CCRC.

Other measures of structural integration and family role occupancy by residential location are provided in Table 5.1. For obvious reasons, residents of congregate housing are more likely to see friends and neighbors almost every day, whereas older residents living in the broader community tend to have more frequent contact with children and other relatives.

Residential group differences in psychological integration are small but significant, with older community residents and CCRC residents feeling the most integrated and shorter term residents of senior housing and movers to the independent/assisted-living complex feeling the least integrated.

PREDICTORS OF STRUCTURAL INTEGRATION

We performed both multiple regression and logistic regression to assess factors related to structural and psychological social integration. The first column of Table 5.2 presents the factors associated with maintaining nonfamily role involvements, in terms of summing up the six nonfamily roles. As we hypothesized, resources are important predictors of structural integration, with the number of limitations on everyday tasks predicting reduced number of role enactments. Seeing relatives more frequently is also associated with maintaining a greater number of nonfamily roles, but being married and caregiving are not. Membership in the older age cohort is marginally related to less nonfamily role involvement.

Residential context matters as well; residents of the CCRC were more likely to maintain or increase their nonfamily roles over the course of the 2-year study. Note that movers to the independent/assisted-living complex also increased their nonfamily role occupancy over time, compared to those who stayed in their own homes within the broader community.

We next estimated the likelihood of maintaining formal volunteering, using logistic regression (column 2 of Table 5.2). Fewer factors are associated with formal volunteering. Having more functional limitations and

TABLE 5.2 Unstandardized Coefficients and Odds Ratios for the Regression of Age Cohort, Gender, Resources, Family Circumstances and Residential Arrangements on Integration in 2000, Controlling for 1998 Integration

	Nonfamily roles[a]			Formal volunteering[b]	Psychological integration[a]		
Resources (1998)							
Education HS or less	—			—	—		
College	−.10	(.13)		.99	-.034	(.041)	
Graduate	.01	(.15)		1.43	-.008	(.048)	
Functional limitations	−.08	(.02)	***	.85***	−.004	(.006)	
Family circumstances (1998)							
Married	−.06	(.11)		.83	.061	(.037)	+
Frequency see relatives	.13	(.04)	**	1.17	.004	(.015)	
Caregiving	.16	(.14)		1.61	-.024	(.046)	
Frequency see children	< .01	(.00)		1.00	< .001	(.000)	
Residential context (2000)							
Community	—			—	—		
Long-term SH	.26	(.17)		.88	-.064	(.057)	
Short-term SH	.29	(.19)		1.10	-.128	(.063)	*
CCRC resident	.63	(.14)	***	1.14	-.099	(.048)	*
Mover to IAL	.45	(.19)	*	.95	-.170	(.066)	*
Age and gender							
Age cohort							
Age 70–79	—	—		—			
Age 80–100	-.28	(.10)	*	.50**	-.030	(.035)	
Female	-.01	(.10)		1.16	.027	(.037)	
1998 Integration							
Multiple roles 1998	.54	(.04)	***				
Formal volunteer 1998				5.81***			
Structural Integration, 1998							
Employed					.074	(.051)	
Community participation							
Formal volunteer					.069	(.042)	+
Informal volunteer					.060	(.050)	
Organization member					.039	(.050)	
No participation					—		
Frequency religious services					.040	(.019)	*
Frequency see neighbors					.048	(.016)	**
Frequency see friends					.022	(.018)	
Psychological integration, 1998					.341	(.040)	***
n	485			479	461		
R-squared	.46			—	.27		

+ p <.10; * p < .05; ** p < .01; *** p < .001.

[a]   Unstandardized coefficients and standard deviations.

[b]   Odds ratios.

CCRC, continuing care retirement community; IAL, independent/assisted living; SH, senior housing.

being in the older age cohort make formal volunteering less likely. Having more education (particularly a graduate education) predicts a higher likelihood of formal volunteering (results not shown), but predicts no change in participation over time. CCRC residents are more likely than older residents living in the community to formally volunteer, but residence does not explain change in participation.

PSYCHOLOGICAL INTEGRATION

We hypothesized that individual resources and family circumstances would be positively related to psychological integration in the form of feeling connected (the Social Integration subscale of the Cutrona Social Provisions Scale). We also postulated that older people living in their own individual homes would be more apt to feel integrated compared to those living in (or having recently moved into) group living arrangements.

Another set of hypotheses relate to the mediating effects of structural integration, positing that people who are objectively integrated in social roles and relationships will perceive themselves as being psychologically integrated as well (see Figure 5.1). At the bivariate level, we find various measures of structural integration are indeed correlated with psychological integration (volunteer $r = .21$, religious participant $r = .22$, club member $r = .20$). Accordingly, we hypothesized that any links between residential location (and possibly resources) and psychological integration would diminish once we include in the model various measures of structural integration (number of nonfamily roles versus particular role involvements). The results are presented in column 3 of Table 5.2. We find little change in the relationship of individual resources, age, and family circumstances to psychological integration, even controlling for various measures of structural integration. However, residential context is more significant when including measures of structural integration. In this model, all those in senior housing for a period of 5 years or less (shorter term residents of senior housing, CCRC residents, and movers to the independent/assisted-living complex) tend to show lower psychological integration than older community residents. Formal volunteering, attending religious services more frequently, and seeing neighbors more frequently are all associated with maintaining feelings of psychological integration.

We also estimated models for women alone by looking at the relationship between marriage and structural and psychological integration. We found a significant interaction between being married and the neighbor role. Specifically, being neighborly (seeing neighbors regularly) is not associated with maintaining psychological integration for married women (results not shown). But it is important for nonmarried women, suggesting the growing significance of relations with neighbors for older women who are not married or who have lost their husbands. All other forms of structural integration (employment, community participation, attending religious services, seeing friends) are important for the psychological integration of older women, regardless of marital status.

CONCLUSION

There is a considerable body of research linking structural and psychological social integration with well-being. Studies have found that integration into society, in terms of multiple role occupancy, reduces the likelihood of psychological distress among both men and women (Gore & Mangione, 1983; Kandel, Davies, & Raveis, 1985; Moen, 1996; Spreitzer, Snyder & Larson, 1979; Thoits, 1983, 1986), and similar findings also link multiple roles to physical health (Moen, Dempster-McClain, & Williams, 1992; Nathanson, 1980, 1984; Verbrugge, 1983, 1985), coronary heart disease (Haynes, Feinleib, Devine, Scotch, & Kannel, 1978; Reed, McGee, & Yano, 1983), and duration of life (Blazer, 1982; House, Robbins, & Metzner, 1982; Moen, Dempster-McClain, & Williams, 1989; Seeman, Kaplan, Knudsen, Cohen, & Guralnik, 1987). There is also a body of research addressing the significance of employment and formal volunteering for psychological integration and well-being (Moen & Fields, 1999; Moen et al., 2000; Moen, Dempster-McClain, & Williams, 1989, 1992).

What is not known are the biographical pathways that promote or detract from being and feeling connected in later adulthood. In this chapter we have examined residential location not as a static ecological address but as a process of transition, a key transition for many older Americans. To do so we compared and contrasted recent movers as opposed to long-term residents in various arrangements. One's residential circumstances can itself indicate location in the social structure in the later years, reflecting a lifetime of cumulation of advantage or disadvantage.

Our findings point to differences in the factors associated with structural integration (actual role occupancy) versus those associated with psychological integration (feeling integrated). For example, declines in health (in terms of increased functional limitations) and simply being in an older age cohort predict less structural integration but not less psychological integration. Being married helps older people feel psychologically integrated but is not associated with their structural integration in terms of actually occupying various roles, perhaps because married older people may not be as motivated to seek social contact outside their family.

Where older people live and for how long also matters for both structural and psychological integration, but in different ways. Residents of senior housing, in particular the CCRC, are not disadvantaged compared to older community residents in terms of the roles they occupy (structural integration). If anything, they tend to have an advantage. Even those who moved most recently (to the independent/assisted-living complex) tended to increase the number of nonfamily roles they occupied after they moved. However, whether or not people feel connected (psychological integration) does appear to be disrupted by relocation. Having moved within the past 5 years to senior housing seems to be a disadvantage for psychological integration. We know that both types of integration—objective and subjective—matter for health and well-being. But our results suggest they are not the same thing. Residential relocation may even facilitate the actual participation of older Americans in their communities. But sustaining or fostering a sense of psychological integration among movers to congregate housing may be more difficult to achieve.

IMPLICATIONS FOR PRACTITIONERS

The findings in this chapter suggest that psychological integration, a sense of belonging, does not necessarily follow from social activities, and may even be relatively independent of social activities for some people. (See also chapter 4.) This raises the question of the accuracy of self-reports of social participation. Research suggests that perceptions of involvement may not necessarily reflect objective social involvement (House, Umberson, & Landis, 1988; Wethington & Kessler, 1986), raising interesting issues for professionals who serve aging populations. How can we foster feelings of belonging if social participation alone is not enough?

The findings here suggest some strategies for encouraging psychological integration. The importance to psychological integration of seeing neighbors frequently may provide an impetus to design physical spaces that maximize opportunities for informal visiting. This may be particularly important for those who are otherwise unlikely to join groups or volunteer. These informal social contacts tend to happen more frequently in senior housing where older people are in closer proximity.

Helping people to maintain attendance at their home religious congregations may also help foster a sense of belonging, when it is geographically possible. For those who have relocated to new areas and for those who have become less mobile, facilitating church attendance on site or in local congregations may foster greater perceived social integration.

Our results also showed that nonfamily role participation was related to feelings of psychological integration for nonmarried women, but not for married women. This suggests that nonfamily roles such as that of neighbor may help promote a feeling of belonging for those who have lost a key family role. Conversely, it may suggest that nonfamily roles are not as important for those who still have a spouse.

These challenges face those working with elders in the community as well as those working within facilities. However, these results show that fostering social integration can start with straightforward solutions, such as giving neighbors opportunities to get involved and helping religious congregation connect with older people. In these situations everyone, not just the older person, wins by strengthening their social connections.

REFERENCES

Aneshensel, C. S., & Frerichs, R. R. (1982). Stress, support, and depression: A longitudinal causal model. *Journal of Community Psychology, 10,* 363–376.

Berkman, L. F., & Breslow, L. (1983). *Health and ways of living: The Alameda County Study.* New York: Oxford University.

Blazer, D. G. (1982). Social support and mortality in an elderly community population. *American Journal of Epidemiology, 115,* 684–694.

Bronfenbrenner, U. (1995). The bioecological model from a life course perspective: Reflections of a patient observer. In P. Moen, G. H. Elder, Jr., K. Luscher (Eds.), *Examining lives in context: Perspectives on the ecology of human development* (pp. 599–618). Washington, DC: American Psychological Association.

Brown, G. W., & Harris, T. (1978). *Social Origins of Depression.* New York: Free.

Cutrona, C., & Russell, D. (1987). The provisions of social relationships and adaptations to stress. In W. H. Jones & D. Perlman (Eds.), *Advances in personal relationships* (Vol. 1, pp. 37–67). Greenwich, CT: JAI.

Durkheim, E. (1951). *Suicide: A study in sociology.* (J. A. Spaulding & G. Simpson, Trans.). New York: Free. (Original work published 1897).

Elder, G. H., Jr., George, L. K., & Shanahan, M. J. (1996). Psychosocial stress over the life course. In H. B. Kaplan (Ed.), *Psychosocial stress: Perspectives on structure, theory, life course, and methods* (pp. 247–291). Orlando, FL: Academic.

Erickson, M. A., Dempster-McClain, D., Whitlow, C., & Moen, P. (2000). Social integration and the move to a continuing care retirement community. In K. Pillemer, P. Moen, E. Wethington, & N. Glasgow (Eds.), *Social integration in the second half of life* (pp. 211–227). Baltimore: Johns Hopkins University.

Folts, W. E., & Yeatts, D. E. (1995). *Housing and the aging population: Options for the new century.* New York: Garland.

Gore, S., & Mangione, T. (1983). Social roles, sex roles, and psychological distress: Additive and interactive models of sex differences. *Journal of Health and Social Behavior, 24*, 300–312.

Gove, W. R., & Geerken, M. R. (1977). The effect of children and employment on the mental health of married men and women. *Social Forces, 56*, 66–76.

Haynes, S. G., Feinleib, M., Devine, S., Scotch, N., & Kannel, W. B. (1978). The relationship of psychosocial factors to coronary heart disease in the Framingham study. *American Journal of Epidemiology, 107*, 384–402.

Herzog, A. R., House, J. S., & Morgan, J. M. (1991). Relation to work and retirement to health and well-being in older age. *Psychology and Aging, 6*, 202–211.

House, J. S., & Kahn, R. L. (1985). Measures and concepts of social support. In S. Cohen & S. L. Syme (Eds.), *Social Support and Health*. New York: Academic.

House, J. S., Robbins, C., & Metzner, H. L. (1982). The association of social relationships and activities with mortality: Prospective evidence from the Tecumseh Community Health Study. *American Journal of Epidemiology, 166*, 123–140.

House, J. S., Umberson, D., & Landis, K. R. (1988). Structures and processes of social support. *Annual Review of Sociology, 14*, 293–318.

Kandel, D., Davies, M., & Raveis, V. (1985). The stressfulness of daily social roles for women: Marital, occupational, and household roles. *Journal of Health and Social Behavior, 26*, 64–78.

Kessler, R. C., & McRae, J. A. (1982). The effect of wives' employment on the mental health of men and women. *American Sociological Review, 27*, 216–227.

Lee, B. A., Oropesa, R. S., & Kanan, J. W. (1994). Neighborhood context and residential mobility. *Demography, 31*, 249–270.

Liang, J, Dvorkin, L., Kahana, E., & Mazian, F. (1980). Social integration and morale: A re-examination. *Journal of Gerontology, 35*, 746–757.

Linton, R. (1936). *The Study of Men*. New York: Appleton Century.

Litwak, E., Messeri, P., Wolfe, S., Gorman, S, Silverstein, M., & Guilarte, M. (1989). Organizational theory, social supports, and mortality rates: A theoretical convergence. *American Sociological Review, 54*(1), 49–66.

Mancini, J. A., & Blieszner, R. (1992). Social provisions in adulthood: Concept and measurement in close relationships. *Journal of Gerontology: Psychological Sciences, 47*(1), 14–20.

Merton, R. K. (1968). *Social theory and social structure*. New York: Free.

Moen, P. (1995). A life course approach to post-retirement roles and well-being. In L. A. Bond, S. J. Cutler, & A. E. Grams (Eds.), *Promoting successful and productive aging* (pp. 239–256). Newbury Park, CA: Sage.

Moen, P. (1996). A life course perspective on retirement, gender, and well-being. *Journal of Occupational Health Psychology, 1*, 131–144.

Moen, P. (2001). The gendered life course. In L. George & R. H. Binstock (Eds.), *Handbook of aging and the social sciences*, (5th Ed., pp. 179–196). San Diego, CA: Academic.

Moen, P., Dempster-McClain, D., & Williams, R. M., Jr. (1989). Social integration and longevity: An event history analysis of women's roles and resilience. *American Sociological Review, 54,* 635–647.

Moen, P., Dempster-McClain, D., & Williams, R. M., Jr. (1992). Successful aging: A life course perspective on women's roles and health. *American Journal of Sociology, 97*(6), 1612–1638.

Moen, P., & Erickson, M. A. (2001). Decision-making and satisfaction with a continuing care retirement community. *Journal of Housing for the Elderly, 14,* 53–69.

Moen, P., & Fields, V. (1999, August). *Retirement and well-being: Does community participation replace paid work?* Paper presented at the American Sociological Association, 94th Annual Meeting, Chicago.

Moen, P., Fields, V., Meador, R., & Rosenblatt, H. (2000). Fostering integration: A case study of the Cornell Retirees Volunteering In Service (CRVIS). In K. Pillemer, P. Moen, E. Wethington, & N. Glasgow (Eds.), *Social integration in the second half of life* (pp. 247–264). Baltimore: Johns Hopkins University.

Musick, M. A., Herzog, A. R., & House, J. S. (1999). Volunteering and mortality among older adults: Findings from a national sample. *Journal of Gerontology: Social Sciences, 54B,* S173–S180.

Nathanson C. (1980). Social roles and health status among women: The significance of employment. *Social Science and Medicine, 14,* 463–471.

Nathanson, C. (1984). Sex differences in mortality. In R. H. Turner & J. F. Short, Jr. (Eds.), *Annual review of sociology,* (Vol. 10, pp. 191–213). Palo Alto, CA: Annual Reviews.

O'Rand, A. (1996). The precious and the precocious: Understanding cumulative disadvantage and cumulative advantage over the life course. *The Gerontologist, 36,* 230–238

Pillemer, K., Moen, P., Wethington, E., & Glasgow, N. (2000). (Eds.). *Social integration in the second half of life.* Baltimore: Johns Hopkins University.

Reed, D., McGee, D., & Yano, K. (1983). Psychosocial processes and general susceptibility to chronic disease. *American Journal of Epidemiology, 119,* 356–370.

Riley, M. W., & Riley, Jr., J. W. (1994). Structural lag: Past in future? In M. W. Riley, R. L. Kahn, & A. Foner (Eds.), *Age and structural lag: The mismatch between people's lives and opportunities in work, family, and leisure.* New York: Wiley.

Rosow, I. (1967). *Social integration of the aged.* New York: Free.

Seeman, T. E., Kaplan, G. A., Knudsen, L., Cohen, R., & Guralnik, J. (1987). Social network ties and mortality among the elderly in the Alameda County Study. *American Journal of Epidemiology, 126*(4), 714–723.

Spreitzer, E., Snyder, E. E., & Larson, D. L. (1979). Multiple roles and psychological well-being. *Sociological Focus, 12,* 141–148.

Thoits, P. A. (1983). Multiple identities and psychological well-being: A reformulation and test of the social isolation hypothesis. *American Sociological Review, 48,* 174–187.

Thoits, P. A. (1986). Multiple identities: Examining gender and marital status differences in distress. *American Sociological Review, 51,* 259–272.

Verbrugge, L. M. (1983). Multiple roles and physical health of women and men. *Journal of Health and Social Behavior, 24,* 16–30.

Verbrugge, L. M. (1985). Gender and health: An update on hypotheses and evidence. *Journal of Health and Social Behavior, 26,* 156–182.

Wethington, E., & Kessler, R. C. (1986). Perceived support, received support, and adjustment to stressful life events. *Journal of Health and Social Behavior, 27,* 78–89.

Williams, R. M., Jr. (1965). *American society: A sociological interpretation.* New York: Knopf.

Young, F. M., & Glasgow, N. (1998). Voluntary social participation and health. *Research on Aging, 20,* 339–362.

SECTION 4

Service Utilization, Health, and Well-Being

CHAPTER 6

Housing, Health, and Disability

Heidi Holmes, Katherine Beissner,
Kelly Welsh, and John A. Krout

D isability among older adults is increasing in prevalence (Dunlop, Manheim, & Chang, 1999; Peek & Coward, 2000), but declining in rate compared to 20 years ago (Manton & Gu, 2001). As people age, disability levels tend to increase and health care providers are challenged with disability prevention and management in this growing segment of society. In many cases, chronic health conditions lead to disability. Health status and chronic disease are impacted by a variety of factors, such as age, genetics, lifestyle, and diet. While age and genetics are not under the control of individuals or health care providers, lifestyle and diet may be. Where people live may also be a factor in their health status. For example, researchers have found that older adults living in rural areas generally suffer from more chronic conditions and have more functional limitations than their urban counterparts (Coward & Krout, 1998). Research has also shown that these health differences cannot be explained simply by variation in the characteristics of rural and urban elders, such as age, gender, race, and income (Gillanders, Buss, & Hofstetter, 1996).

Thus, factors related to where older people live such as lifestyle patterns, including exercise and diet, availability of health services, and types of employment, can be expected to influence health status. We can also speculate that the type of housing older people live in may affect health. Housing that does not match functional abilities (for those with impairments such as mobility difficulties) exposes older adults to environmental stresses (Lawton & Nahemow, 1973). Congregate housing that includes services such as meals provided under the supervision of a nutritionist or has safety features such as call bells or ADA compliment bathroom fixtures may both prevent and/or delay health conditions or disease from becoming disabling conditions, and help in the management of disabilities.

The *Pathways to Life Quality* study provides an opportunity to examine whether and how the type of housing older adults live in affects the relationships among factors that have been found to influence health conditions and rates of disability. This chapter seeks to answer the following questions:

- What are the relationships between disease, disability, and housing?
- What role do demographics, functional limitations, and health behaviors play in the development of various chronic illnesses?
- How do the various chronic illnesses and health behaviors contribute to disability?

HEALTH AND HOUSING

The increase in life expectancy has meant that older adults are living more years in their own homes. Many of these older adults choose to stay in environments that may not match their functional abilities or needs, and consequently invoke both informal and formal support systems—help from children and home care, respectively. Greater numbers of older adults are living in settings that have a variety of support systems in place so as to allow for more independent living, such as assisted-living residences and continuing care retirement communities (CCRCs). However, researchers have rarely looked at how these living environments impact residents' health status, disability progression, or ability to remain independent. A number of factors have been shown by previous research to affect health and disability. These include diet and obesity, exercise, alcohol consumption, and smoking. While researchers have examined differences between rural and urban areas (Coward & Krout, 1998), virtually no research has examined differences in health on the basis of the type of environments in which older people live.

Many researchers classify their subjects as disabled when they no longer live independently, but live in an institutional setting (Dunlop et al., 1999; Fuchs et al., 1998). For example, Dunlop and colleagues investigated successful aging in an older population by looking at chronic illnesses, limitations, and disabilities. Interestingly, living in the community independently was considered successful and moving to a nursing home or receiving in-home care for 3 months or more was considered unsuccessful. Thus, studies of health and aging often exclude those living in assisted-living residences or other forms of congregate housing. Further confounding the study of the relationship between housing and health is the fact that a high proportion of senior citizens with chronic health conditions that could be considered disabled live in communities with the help of informal or home care supports. These support systems often allow people to remain at home rather than having to move to nursing homes. The U.S. Census Bureau (1997) reports that 4.4 million older adults living in noninstitutional settings require assistance with one or more activities of daily living (ADLs).

Research on nursing home residents has shown that some of their disabilities are related to the lack of opportunities for exercise and social interaction in those environments (Fiatarone, 1996). Obviously, people who go to nursing homes in the first place have significant chronic impairments and are likely to become more impaired over time. However, the nursing home environment itself can either accelerate or slow down decline, depending on the type of activities and treatments that are made available. Although much of the impact of nursing homes is a result of staffing, resources, and philosophy, the physical environment itself creates some the effects.

The *Pathways* study does not include nursing home residents, but it does include a variety of housing environments, such as congregate housing and single-family dwelling units in the greater community. This range of living arrangements allows us to identify specific antecedents of health and well-being that may be affected by living in congregate housing. For example, some congregate housing settings have on-site staff or receive expertise from off-site staff in preparing meals and providing recreation, exercise, or health-promotion activities. Other congregate housing settings for seniors do not. We investigate residential differences in the health behaviors, chronic conditions and illnesses, and rates of disability that have been reported by the *Pathways to Life Quality* study.

HEALTH BEHAVIORS, CHRONIC CONDITIONS, RISK FACTORS, AND DISABILITIES

HEALTH BEHAVIORS AND CHRONIC CONDITIONS

The health behaviors of older adults play an integral role in the development of chronic illnesses, which often lead to disability. A considerable body of research has examined the impact of specific chronic conditions on functional decline and disability in older adults through both cross-sectional and longitudinal studies.

Diet and Obesity

Diet influences obesity and coronary heart disease (Stare & Whelan, 1990). Obesity, in turn, is associated with numerous chronic conditions including diabetes, stroke, hypertension, and coronary heart disease (CHD). Research has shown that there is a relationship between hip fractures and high body mass index (BMI) scores. High BMI scores are indicative of obesity. Prior research on the impact of obesity on disability has shown mixed results. Guralnik and Kaplan (1989) found that normal weight predicts higher levels of function, while Visser and colleagues (1998) found that high body fatness was associated with mobility-related disability and that fat mass predicts disability. Peek and Coward (2000) found that obesity carries a 2.1 times higher risk of limitations in performing the ADLs, and a 1.39 times increased risk of limitations in performing the instrumental activities of daily living (IADLs), while Cho and colleagues (1998) found that baseline obesity was not associated with decline in performance of the ADLs in 3 years. Where a person lives or the housing environment of an older individual may impact diet and obesity because many senior housing facilities provide congregate meals prepared by dieticians and may offer special meals to those with specific health conditions or concerns.

Exercise

Research has also shown exercise to impact the development of conditions. Persons participating in medium- to high-intensity exercise routines have the greatest relief of arthritis pain and disability, control over type 2 diabetes, lowered risk of CHD, lowered existing blood pressure, and risk of hypertension reduced by 50% (Rowe & Kahn, 1997; Wannamethee, Shaper, Gerald, George, & Alberti, 2000). Moderate to intense exercise also reduces an individual's risk of ischemic stroke (Hu, Stampfer, Colditz, & Ascherio 2000; Krohn & LoBuono, 2000). Physical activity can slow or stop the progression of pulmonary, musculoskeletal, and metabolic-endocrine changes, while physical inactivity leads to osteoporosis and decreased muscle strength (Laukkanen, Kauppinen, & Heikkinen, 1998). Residents of senior housing may experience increased incentives and opportunities to exercise compared to community-dwelling residents. Many senior housing facilities are being built with recreation or exercise rooms. The more sophisticated CCRCs often have onsite occupational or physical therapists and recreation staff to assist residents with exercise programs and rehabilitative exercise regimens. However, lower income senior apartments may not offer these opportunities.

Smoking

Research shows that smoking also impacts the development of chronic conditions. The Centers for Disease Control (1994) issued a report concerning the influence of various risk factors on the prevalence of chronic conditions. Results showed smoking, obesity, and a sedentary lifestyle play a crucial role in the development of chronic conditions. Individuals with fewer than 12 years of education were more likely to possess these risk factors. Smoking greatly influences the development of lung disease, including chronic obstructive pulmonary disease (emphysema) and lung cancer (Pace, 2000). Levangie (1999) found a strong correlation between smoking and increased occurrence of musculoskeletal problems. However, cigarette smoking has a decreased impact on the development of CHD as one becomes older (Beaglehole, 1991; Benfante & Reed, 1990). Of the senior housing facilities participating in the *Pathways* study, only one—the government-subsidized public housing—allows smoking in the common areas of the building, and even these buildings are increasingly becoming smoke free.

HEALTH CONDITIONS AND DISABILITY

We are not aware of any research into how housing affects the link between health condition and disability. We speculate that the housing environments with more services and programs may reduce the disability associated with some conditions, such as diabetes and arthritis. While research shows distinct relationships between chronic conditions and disability, it is difficult to determine how housing relates to these incidences.

Arthritis

Because of the prevalence of arthritic conditions, this condition has been particularly well studied. People with arthritis have greater need in all aspects of disablement, including physical function, personal care, and household management (Verbrugge, Lepkowski, & Konkol, 1991). When considering comorbidities, those who had arthritis and other chronic conditions had higher disability levels than those with arthritis alone or other chronic conditions. Stewart and colleagues (1989) also found that arthritic conditions predisposed persons to broad ranges of disability.

Peek and Coward (2000) found that persons with self-reported arthritis had an increased risk of decline in the ability to perform the ADLs and the IADLs as compared to those without arthritis. Boult, Kane, Louis, Boult & McCaffrey (1994) substantiate these findings in a longitudinal study that showed that self-reported arthritis predicted functional limitations at a 4-year follow-up.

Cardiovascular Diseases and Hypertension

Another prevalent condition affecting older adults is heart disease, including general coronary artery disease, myocardial infarction, congestive heart failure, and angina. Guccione and colleagues (1994) found that heart disease was associated with disability in performing four of seven functional tasks. Peek and Coward (2000) found increased risk of both ADL and IADL disability for those with heart disease. Interestingly, Boult and colleagues (1994) found that coronary artery disease was not predictive of functional limitation at a 4-year follow-up.

A related but separate condition, hypertension, has received some consideration in the literature on disability. Cho and colleagues (1998) found that baseline hypertension was associated with a decline in the performance of the ADLs 3 years later, and Guralnik and Kaplan (1989) found the absence of hypertension was predictive of higher levels of functioning.

Diabetes

Persons with self-reported diabetes have been found to have lower functional levels as well as lower health perceptions than patients without diabetes (Stewart et al., 1989). Other researchers found that those with diabetes were more likely to experience functional decline by a 2-year follow-up date (Mor et al., 1989). Peek and Coward (2000) found increased risk for ADL and IADL limitations in those with diabetes, while Kaplan (1991) found an association between diabetes and mobility disability. For seniors living in senior housing with on-site meals, dietary oversight may help to delay the progression of disability for those with this condition. Many independent-living apartment complexes with congregate dining offer menu selections for diabetics. The dietary staff may provide these meals, but ultimately it is up to the residents to make their own food choices.

Cerebrovascular Disease

Researchers investigating the impact of stroke or other cerebrovascular conditions on disability have found strong associations between stroke and disability (Campbell, Busby, Robertson, Langlois, & Morgan, 1994; Kelly-Hayes, Jette, Wolf, D'Agostino, & O'Dell, 1992; Mor et al., 1989; Peek & Coward, 2000). Barret-Conner and Wingard (1991) found that men who had a history of stroke had increased risk for dependency, but this increased risk was not seen in female stroke survivors. Jette, Pinsky, Branch, Wolf, and Feinleib (1988) found that a history of stroke was the strongest predictor of disability when controlling for age, other cardiovascular disease, and cardiovascular risk factors.

Orthopedic Conditions

Orthopedic conditions have significant effects on the function of older adults. Bergstrom and colleagues (1985) found that limitations in range of motion in hip and knee were associated with difficulty in performing select activities, and decreased hip mobility was associated with the need for ambulation assistance. Persons with low back pain were found to have decreased physical function and role function, higher levels of bodily pain, and lower health perceptions than those without back problems (Stewart et al., 1989). Older women with severe back pain showed increased difficulty in mobility and in performing the ADLs, but not the inability to perform these tasks (Leveille, Guralnik, Hochber, & Hirsch, 1999). Given these research findings, mobility-related disability would seem to be the primary concern for those who are thinking of relocating, making modifications to the house, or contracting outside services. Mobility impairments, as well as other potentially disabling health conditions, are included in our analyses.

RESEARCH QUESTIONS

Given the research on housing, health behaviors, chronic conditions and illnesses, and disability, we used the *Pathways to Life Quality* data to examine the following questions:

- What are the relationships between health behaviors, chronic conditions, disability, and housing?
- What roles do demographics, functional limitations, and health behaviors play in the development of various chronic illnesses?
- How do the various chronic illnesses and health behaviors contribute to disability?

METHODOLOGICAL ISSUES

The *Pathways* data we used to investigate these questions were from 687 individuals who were interviewed at both time 1 (1997–1998) and time 2 (1999–2000). In this sample, three of five (59%) lived in their own homes in the greater community, referred to hereafter as *the community sample*, and 41% lived in senior housing. The two types were grouped into a three-level dummy variable: those who resided in their own homes within the greater community; those who lived in one of the various independent-living senior-apartment complexes that have few (if any) on-site services; and those who resided in service-rich retirement communities such as a CCRC or an independent/assisted-living facility (not including nursing homes).

SAMPLE DEMOGRAPHIC

The community sample was randomly selected from those older than 60 living in the county. The demographics of the random sample closely matched those of the county (Henderson & Oggins, 1999). The facilities samples are convenience samples of those willing to participate in the study. Approximately half of the residents of the service-rich retirement community chose to participate in the study. Of the senior-apartment residents, one half to less than one quarter of all residents agreed to participate. Table 6.1 shows the demographic composition of the community and the facilities samples. Chi-square analysis was used to assess differences in the marital status ($X^2 = 103.13$, $df = 2$, $p < .001$) and education levels ($X^2 = 79.29$, $df = 2$, $p < .001$) of the residents of the community and the senior housing facilities. Many more community residents were married than were residents of the service-rich retirement community, and senior apartments. Education levels also varied, with retirement-community residents and community residents having higher percentages of college or advanced degrees than senior-apartment residents.

MEASURES

The interview items we analyzed included questions on the respondents' health conditions, self-assessed health on a scale of 0 (worst possible health) to 10 (best possible health), frequency and type of exercise, dietary changes, smoking history, height and weight, age, and activity limitations. Height and weight were transformed into a BML score for each respondent and this score was used in subsequent analyses. The most prevalent health con-

TABLE 6.1 Demographic Characteristics of the *Pathways to Life Quality* Sample

	Community	Service-rich	Service-poor
Age	74	80	78
Gender	66% women	64% women	85% women
	34% men	36% men	15% men
Income	$47,970	$74,400	$15,600
Married	52%	54%	10%
College/graduate education	75%	93%	47%
Children	3	3	3
Employed	17%	10%	3%

ditions in our sample that could be impacted by behavior included hypertension (34%), heart conditions (21%), arthritis (12%), diabetes (8%), musculoskeletal conditions (8%), lung conditions (7%), osteoporosis (4%), and stroke (3%). Few respondents reported cancer incidence, and this condition was excluded from analysis.

Two items concerning exercise were included in the analyses. The first variable consisted of the frequency of exercise per week, and the second was a list of the most frequent exercises. The most vigorous exercises were summed into an aerobic exercise variable. These exercises included brisk walking/hiking, calisthenics/aerobics, cycling, running/jogging, swimming, and racquet sports. While 35% did not engage in vigorous exercise, 59% participated in one or two of these exercises.

Items on respondents' activity limitations were entered into factor analysis with varimax rotation in order to determine categories of limitations or disability. The factor analysis yielded no specific categories for items in either the first or the second interview. We then took select items as indicators of disability and created a summed disability score for the second-wave interview responses. The disability variable included difficulty in walking six blocks; climbing a flight of stairs; doing day-to-day household tasks; caring for personal needs (dressing, eating, toileting); moving about inside the house; and bending, kneeling, or stooping. This disability variable was used as the dependent variable in linear regression analysis, with all of the wave-2 health conditions, wave-1 health behavior variables, and wave-1 demographics as predictors.

FINDINGS

Our first two questions were What are the relationships between health behaviors, chronic conditions, disability, and housing? and What role do demographics, functional limitations, and health behaviors play in the development of various chronic conditions? Analysis of variance tests were used to test for differences in the health behavior variables, disability scores, and age among the respondents in the various living arrangements (Table 6.2). Significant differences were seen in the ages of respondents in all of the living arrangements, and between the community sample and congregate housing residents' levels of disability and activity limitations. Community-dwelling residents were younger (average age 74) than senior-apartment residents (average age 78), and the senior-apartment residents were younger than the service-rich retirement community residents (average age 80). Functional limitations were lower in the sample from the community (.68) than in the sample from those in apartments (1.61) and service-rich retirement communities (1.12). Disability rates were higher in the service-rich retirement community (1.13) and senior apartments (1.35) than in the community (.59).

Overall, the residents of senior apartments had poorer health behaviors than the other groups. They engaged in fewer intense exercises (.54) than community (.89) and service-rich retirement community (1.07) residents. As measured by BMI scores, they are also more obese (26.8) than community (25.3) and service-rich retirement community (24.7) residents. They stopped smoking at an older age (55) than did the residents of the other two groups (46). Similarly, senior-apartment residents consumed fewer alcoholic beverages (44.5) per year than did residents in the community (127) and the service-rich retirement community (138).

To answer the question on relationships between health behaviors, chronic conditions, disability, and housing, we conducted independent samples t-tests and chi-square analyses. These analyses assessed differences between those with and without each of the illnesses on demographics (W1), living arrangement, and the aforementioned health behavior variables (W1). Table 6.3 presents the results of a linear regression analysis that predicted disability (W2) from health conditions (W2), functional limitations (W1), and health behavior risk variables (W1).

Individuals with heart conditions were older, were older when they quit smoking, engaged in fewer intense exercises, and had significantly more comorbid conditions. They do not differ in frequency of exercise or obesity ratings. The average BMI score for both groups, was 25, indicating

TABLE 6.2 Differences in Health Behaviors, Disability, and Age Among Residents of Different Living Arrangements

	Community (n=407)	Service Rich (n=164)	Service Poor (n=116)
Age[1]	74	80	78
Number of Intense Exercises[2]	.89	1.07	.54
Body mass index[3]	25.3	24.7	26.8
Alcoholic drinks per year[4]	127	138	45
Age stopped smoking[5]	46	46	55
Disability score[6]	.59	1.13	1.35
Functional Limitations[7]	.68	1.12	1.61

[1] $F = 48.99$, df = 2,676, $p \leq .001$
[2] $F = 11.73$, df = 2,609, $p \leq .001$
[3] $F = 6.72$, df = 2,662, $p \leq .001$
[4] $F = 12.19$, df = 2,673, $p \leq .001$
[5] $F = 8.68$, df = 2,300, $p \leq .001$
[6] $F = 17.13$, df = 2,654, $p \leq .001$
[7] $F = 28.97$, df = 2,675, $p \leq .001$

that our respondents were in the healthy range. Respondents with hypertension had higher BMI scores and more comorbid conditions. Those having suffered a stroke were older and had a greater number of comorbid conditions.

Respondents with gastrointestinal difficulties ceased smoking at an older age. Those with diabetes had higher BMI scores, stopped smoking at an older age, exercised less often, participated in fewer intense exercises, and had more comorbid conditions. Respondents reporting lung conditions were older when they stopped smoking, exercise less often, and had more comorbid conditions. Respondents with arthritis engaged in fewer intense exercises and had more comorbid conditions. Similarly, those with musculoskeletal impairments had higher comorbidity rates.

Our last research question asked How do the various chronic illnesses and health behaviors contribute to disability? The linear regression model for disability yielded the following predictors: housing type, intense exercise, stroke incidence, and recent dietary changes. Those with higher disability scores had higher rates of stroke, had reported dietary changes at wave 1, engaged in fewer high-intensity exercises, and were more likely to live in service-rich senior housing. The results are shown in Table 6.4.

TABLE 6.3 Differences in the Predisposing Disease Risk Factors by Chronic Condition

	With		Without			
Factor	M	sd	M	sd	df	t
Heart						
Age quit smoking	51.35	15.26	46.72	13.83	301	−2.38**
Age	76.45	7.25	73.29	7.68	683	−4.52***
Intense exercise	.65	.75	.94	.86	610	3.47***
Comorbidities	2.04	.92	.75	.90	684	−15.50***
Hypertension						
Body mass	26.10	4.63	25.08	4.57	666	−2.71**
Comorbidities	1.81	.91	.64	.89	684	−15.96***
Diabetes						
Body Mass	28.04	5.98	25.20	4.42	53	−3.28**
Age quit smoking	53.60	15.71	47.25	14.05	301	−2.14*
Exercise frequency	3.71	2.98	4.82	2.76	60	2.62**
Intense exercise	.43	.68	.91	.84	610	3.59***
Comorbidities	2.37	.98	.92	.98	684	−10.50***
Lung disease						
Age quit smoking	53.67	16.79	47.13	13.85	33	−2.06*
Exercise frequency	3.88	2.82	4.79	2.78	676	2.21*
Comorbidities	2.27	.94	.94	1.00	684	−8.94***
Musculoskeletal disease						
Comorbidities	2.62	1.05	0.89	0.93	62	−1.73***
Gastrointestinal						
Age quit smoking	54.15	12.87	47.15	14.27	301	−2.45**
Stroke						
Age	77.94	6.14	73.88	7.71	683	−2.22*
Comorbidities	1.30	1.13	1.00	1.04	684	−2.15*
Arthritis						
Intense exercises	.63	.82	.92	.84	610	2.87***
Comorbidities	2.27	1.04	.86	.94	684	−12.52***

*** $p < .001$; ** $p < .01$; * $p < .05$.

Linear regression analysis of comorbidities controlling for each of the health-risk variables indicated that those with multiple comorbidities had lower levels of education and engaged in fewer intense exercises. It is probable that the illnesses prevent engagement in the more intense exercises.

In order to assess differences in the incidence of each illness by living arrangement, chi-square analyses were used. There were no differences for the majority of the chronic illnesses, with the exception of heart con-

TABLE 6.4 Predictors of Disability and Comorbidities[a]

| | Unstandardized | | | | |
	ß	SE	ß	t	df
Disability					4, 109
Stroke	1.82	.60	.25	3.03**	
Dietary change (T1)	.53	.25	.18	2.14*	
Intense exercises (T1)	−.38	.15	−.26	−2.60**	
Housing type	−.59	.21	−.26	−2.83**	
Comorbidities					2, 116
Education	−.19	.08	−.22	−2.29*	
Intense exercises (T1)	−.27	.13	−.19	−2.11*	

*** $p < .001$; ** $p < .01$; * $p < .05$.
Note: [a] Stepwise linear regression analysis.

ditions ($X^2 = 12.20$, $df = 2$, $p < .01$), hypertension ($X^2 = 7.22$, $df = 2$, $p < .05$), and diabetes ($X^2 = 9.90$, $df = 2$, $p < .01$). Heart disease was more prevalent in the community residents (10.9%) and senior-apartment residents (5.7%) than in the more supportive retirement-community residents (5.3%). Community-dwelling residents (18.2%) had a higher incidence of hypertension than senior-apartment residents (7.5%) and those living in service-rich retirement communities (7.6%). Similarly, diabetes ($X^2 = 9.90$, $df = 2$, $p < .01$) was seen more frequently in community residents (3.5%) and senior-apartment residents (2.5%) than in retirement community residents (1.6%).

IMPLICATIONS FOR RESEARCH, POLICY, AND PRACTICE

Demographics, functional limitations, and health behaviors were found to have relationships to the predominant chronic illnesses reported by respondents in the *Pathways to Life Quality* study. Differences in disease incidence and health behaviors were also seen among the residents of the various housing arrangements. Respondents with multiple chronic health conditions had less education and were likely to be unmarried—both factors for fewer healthful behaviors (Schone & Weinick, 1998). Those with the higher disability scores were those who had suffered stroke, consumed little alcohol, were older when they stopped smoking, and had made recent dietary changes. Although we did not find arthritis or other musculoskeletal impairments to be related to higher rates of disability in this analysis, we may see mobility-related disability increase as we continue to interview our respondents in the coming years.

Chronic conditions reflect the cumulative impact of many factors, such as health behaviors, over many years. They do not result from living for a few years in one setting as opposed to another. Residents living in senior housing have spent many more years living in a variety of nonsenior-housing environments. Thus, our findings do not demonstrate that housing causes the observed chronic conditions. Nonetheless, from practice and policy perspectives, these findings are important because they document the health and disability differences between different housing arrangements and underscore the fact that chronic illness will be found in residents of all types of housing. Thus, treatment, education, and prevention are needed in all of them. An interesting research question is whether or not, over time rates or types of change in chronic conditions differ between housing environments and whether this kind of change is also related to the level of chronic illness residents bring to such housing.

However, we did find a relationship between housing and disability; those having higher levels of disability resided in senior housing environments as opposed to other settings. Senior-apartment (service-poor) residents had the lowest levels of education and income, are typically not married, have poorer health behaviors, and suffer from serious health conditions, such as heart conditions and diabetes. Their disability and functional limitation rates are higher than those of people living in the other environments. The housing complexes in which these residents reside have informal buddy-system networks, but few (if any) have on-site services to enable them to live independently for a longer time. It is evident that these residents are in need of support services and access to social workers or other professionals for linkages to services. Many of the complexes are in more rural areas where home-based services are often difficult to acquire and maintain. Further, budgets for these facilities are often small and they have only part-time on-site managers. Thus, on-site social work support is not possible.

Given these limitations, interesting questions with serious implications for facility managers, policy makers, and health care providers arise: How do the lack of resources and higher rates of illness and disability impact the life quality and mortality rate of these individuals compared to those living in service-rich senior housing? How do varying levels of disability affect the ability of residents to continue to live in their apartments? How can managers change their policies to accommodate residents who are becoming increasingly frail? How can managers assume the role of helping to coordinate services for residents in need?

It is likely that the residents of service-rich environments sought housing where services were available primarily because of health declines. Perhaps these residents were more willing and able to plan ahead for such declines or afford more expensive housing. Thus, we suggest that the housing does not cause the higher levels of disability, but that a selection effect results in more disabled seniors' living in housing with more services. In one sense this suggests a policy success—more disabled elders are found in more supportive living environments.

We also need to ask whether living in service-enriched housing slows the decline in ability. That is, does it have any preventive effect over time? Theoretically, that would be found to be the case. We need to investigate how to provide supportive services that help older adults age more successfully in the environment of their choosing, whether that is a senior apartment, their own home in the community, or a multilevel-care senior housing facility. The *Pathways to Life Quality* study, with its longitudinal focus, should provide us with useful information to answer these questions. This is the strength.

SUMMARY AND CONCLUSIONS

Lifelong patterns of health behavior do appear to impact the development of chronic conditions and to impact disability. It is apparent that those with lower levels of education and poorer economic backgrounds have higher rates of chronic conditions and disability. Many of these frailer older adults have chosen to reside in senior apartments, an arrangement that is more cost-effective, affords them peer companionship, and provides freedom from home maintenance and upkeep. However, it does not necessarily furnish them with a greater service base, and these residents are not in the optimal physical or financial positions to obtain the services they may need. Those with the resources to relocate to service-rich environments also have some serious chronic conditions, yet they have access to a variety of support services, health professionals, and rehabilitative programs. It is probable that the service-rich retirement community residents will be better able to successfully delay disability, provided they make use of these opportunities. By following these older adults over time, we will gain a greater understanding of how housing relates to chronic conditions and disability over time. We will also be able to study which types of supportive programs and resources are most beneficial.

The community-dwelling residents are the healthiest group and are more likely to be married—a factor that often leads to more healthful behaviors and better overall well-being, for men in particular. The demographics of these residents are similar to those of the county from which the sample was drawn; however, this particular county has higher-than-average education and income levels. As we follow them over time, we will be able to track their health behaviors, health conditions, and housing changes. It will be interesting to see how the health-behavior profiles and health conditions of those who move to senior housing match those of the current residents. The answers to these research questions carry with them implications that will be of great importance for housing managers, for those creating long-term care policies, and for service providers.

REFERENCES

Barrett-Conner, E., & Wingard, E. L. (1991). Heart disease risk factors as determinants of dependency and death in an older cohort. *Journal of Aging and Health, 3*, 247–261.

Beaglehole, R. (1991). Coronary heart disease and elderly people. *British Medical Journal, 303*, 69(2), 69–70.

Benfante, R., & Reed, D. (1990). Is elevated serum cholesterol level a risk factor for coronary heart disease in the elderly? *The Journal of the American Medical Association, 263*, 393(4), 393–396.

Bergstrom, G., Aniansson, A., Bjelle, A., Grimby, G., Lundgren-Lindquist, B., & Svanborg, A. (1985). Functional consequences of joint impairment at age 79. *Scandinavian Journal of Rehabilitation Medicine, 17*, 183–190.

Boult, C., Kane, R. L., Louis, T. A., Boult, L., & McCaffrey, D. (1994). Chronic conditions that lead to functional limitation in the elderly. *Journals of Gerontology: Medical Sciences, 49*, M28–M36.

Campbell, A. J., Busby, W. J., Robertson, C. L., Langlois, J. A., & Morgan, F. C. (1994). Disease, impairment, disability and social handicap: A community-based study of people aged 70 years and over. *Disability and Rehabilitation, 16*, 72–79.

Centers for Disease Control (CDC). (1994). Prevalence of selected risk factors for chronic disease by education level in racial/ethnic populations. *U.S. Morbidity and Mortality Weekly Report, 43*(48), 894–899.

Cho, C., Alessi, C. A., Cho, M., Aronow, H. U., Stuck, A. E., Rubenstein, L. Z., & Beck, J. C. (1998). The association between chronic illness and functional change among participants in a comprehensive geriatric assessment program. *Journal of American Geriatrics Society, 46*, 677–682.

Coward, R. T., & Krout, J. A. (1998). *Aging in Rural Settings: Life Circumstances and Distinctive Features.* New York: Springer.

Dunlop, D. D., Manheim, L. M., & Chang, R. W. (1999, August). *Chronic illness, functional limitations, and successful aging.* (AARP Andrus Foundation Report.) Evanston, IL: Institute for Health Services Research and Policy Studies, Northwestern University.

Fiatarone, M. A. (1996). Physical activity and functional independence in aging. *Research Exercise Sport, 67*(3 Suppl.), S70.

Fuchs, Z., Blumstein, T., Novikov, I., Walter-Ginzburg, A., Lyanders, M., Gindin, J., Habot, B., & Modan, B. (1998). Morbidity, comorbidity, and their association with disability among community-dwelling oldest-old in Israel. *Journals of Gerontology: Medical Sciences, 53*(6), M447–M455.

Gillanders, W. R., Buss, T.F., & Hofstetter, C. R. (1996). Urban/rural elderly health status differences: The dichotomy reexamined. *Journal of Aging and Social Policy, 8,* 7–25.

Guccione A. A., Felson D. T., Anderson J. J., Anthony, J. M., Zhang Y., Wilson P. W. F., Kelly-Hayes, M., Wolf, P. A., Kreger B. E., & Kannel, W. B. (1994). The effects of specific medical conditions on the functional limitations of elders in the Framingham Study. *American Journal of Public Health, 84,* 351–358.

Guralnik, J. M., & Kaplan, G. A. (1989). Predictors of healthy aging: Prospective evidence from the Alameda County study. *American Journal of Physical Therapy, 79,* 703–708.

Henderson, C., & Oggins, J. (1999, April). Pathways research and sampling design. *Pathways Working Paper #7.* Cornell University.

Hu, F.B., Stampfer, M. J., Colditz, G. A., & Ascherio, A. (2000). Physical activity and the risk of stroke in women. *The Journal of the American Medical Association, 283,* 2961.

Jette, A. M., Pinsky J. L., Branch L. G., Wolf, P. A., & Feinleib, M. (1988). The Framingham disability study: Physical disability among community-dwelling survivors of stroke. *Journal of Clinical Epidemiology, 69,* 719–726.

Kaplan, G. A. (1991). Epidemiologic observations on the compression of morbidity. *Journal of Aging and Health, 3,* 155–171.

Kelly-Hayes, M., Jette, A. M., Wolf, P. A., D'Agostino, R. B., & O'Dell, P. M. (1992). Functional limitations and disability among elders in the Framingham Study. *American Journal of Public Health, 82,* 841–845.

Krohn, T., & LoBuono, C. (2000). Exercise lowers stroke risk in women. *Patient Care, 34,* 70.

Laukkanen, P., Kauppinen, M., & Heikkinen, E. (1998). Physical activity as a predictor of health and disability in 75- and 80-year-old men and women: A five-year longitudinal study. *Journal of Aging and Physical Activity, 6,* 141–156.

Lawton, M. P., & Nahemow, L. (1973). Ecology and the aging process. In C. Eisdorfer & M. P. Lawton (Eds.), *Psychology of Adult Development and Aging.* Washington, DC: American Psychological Association.

Levangie, P. K. (1999). Association of low back pain with self-reported risk factors among patients seeking physical therapy service. *The Physical Therapy Journal, 79,* 757–765.

Leveille, S. G., Guralnik, J. M., Hochberg, M., & Hirsch, R. (1999). Low back pain and disability in older women: Independent association with difficulty but not inability to perform daily activities. *Journals of Gerontology: Medical Sciences, 54A*, M487–493.

Manton, K. G., & Gu, X. (2001). Changes in the prevalence of chronic disability in the United States black and nonblack population above age 65 from 1982 to 1999. *Proceedings of the National Academy of Sciences, 98*(11), 6354–6359

Mor, V., Murphy, J., Masterson-Allen, S., Willey, C., Razmpour, A., Jackson, M. E., Greer, D., & Katz, S. (1989). Risk of functional decline among well elders. *Journal of Clinical Epidemiology, 42*, 895–904.

Pace, B. (2000). Lung disease. *Journal of the American Medical Association, 283*, 1922.

Peek, M. K., & Coward, R. T. (2000). Antecedents of disability for older adults with multiple chronic health conditions. *Research on Aging, 22*, 422–444.

Rowe, J. W., & Kahn, R. L. (1997). Successful aging. *The Gerontologist, 37*(4), 433–440.

Schone, B. S., & Weinick, R. (1998). Health-related behaviors and the benefits of marriage for elderly persons. *The Gerontologist, 38*(10), 618.

Stare, F. J., & Whelan, E. (1990). Nutrition. *Journal of the American Medical Association, 263*, 2661–2664.

Stewart, A. L., Greenfield, S., Hays, R. D., Wells, K., Rogers, W. H., Berry, S. D., McGlynn, E. A., & Ware, J. E., Jr. (1989). Functional status and well-being of patients with chronic conditions. *Journal of American Medical Association, 262*, 907–913.

U.S. Census Bureau. (1997). *1997 Population profile of the United States: Current population reports special studies P23-194*. U.S. Department of Commerce, Economic and Statistics Administration. Washington DC: U.S. Census Bureau.

Verbrugge, L. M., Lepkowski, J. M., & Konkol, L. L. (1991). Levels of disability among U.S. adults with arthritis. *The Journals of Gerontology: Social Sciences, 16*, S71–S83.

Visser, M., Langlois, J., Harris, T. B., Williamson, J. D., Robbins, J., Kronmal, R. A., Cauley, J. A., & Guralnik, J. M. (1998). High body fatness, but not low fat-free mass, predicts disability in older men and women: The Cardiovascular Health Study. *American Journal of Clinical Nutrition, 68*, 584–590.

Wannamethee, S. G., Shaper, A., Gerald, K., George M. M., & Alberti. (2000). Physical activity, metabolic factors, and the incidence of coronary heart disease and type 2 diabetes. *Archives of Internal Medicine, 160*, 2108.

CHAPTER 7

Utilization of Community-Based Services

Heidi Holmes, John A. Krout, and Sarah Wolle

The majority of care received by older adults is provided by informal supports such as family and friends, even when the older person is frail and requires high levels of care over long periods of time
(Kassner & Bectel, 1998). Nonetheless, formal services play an important
role in meeting the needs of older adults and facilitating independence. It
is estimated that about 20 to 25% of older adults use one or more support
services annually (Biegel, Farkas, & Wadsworth, 1994). While the mix of
formal and informal services depends on the nature of the need, Whitelach
and Noelker (1996) report the following: among disabled older persons in
the United States approximately 20% rely only on formal services; 16%
mix formal and informal care; one third use only informal care; and 29%
receive no assistance. Formal nonmedical services are delivered through
the aging-services network, which consists of close to 30,000 organizations nationwide that provide programs such as congregate meals and social
activities, home care and homemaker services, information and referral,
care management, exercise and health promotion, and transportation
(Wacker, Roberto, & Piper, 1998). However, their utilization is often
impeded by a lack of information, access, and linkages between and to
other community systems (Kim, 1994).

Historically, housing and aging service programs have not been well
integrated or coordinated. Most older adults live in residential settings
(their own homes or senior apartments) where services are not planned or
integrated with the environment. Major exceptions are nursing homes and,
recently, service-rich housing such as independent-living and assisted-living residences and continuing care retirement communities (CCRCs). Many

communities have witnessed the growth of naturally occurring retirement communities (NORCs)—a building, housing development, or neighborhood with a high percentage of older people. NORCs are not planned for this population and usually do not have the health and social services that are needed to maintain independence and meet long-term care needs (Bassuk, 1999). This lack of housing-and-service linkage creates problems in meeting the needs of older adults with chronic health problems and in delivering health-promotion and illness-prevention programs.

While researchers have devoted some attention to studying the patterns and correlates of community-based service utilization, they have generally not looked at how service use changes when older adults move to congregate facilities or how patterns differ for residents of different types of housing. The *Pathways to Life Quality* study allows us to do both because it encompasses older adults from a wide range of living environments, is longitudinal, and has tracked some individuals before and after they have moved. Specifically, we present data to answer the following three questions:

- What is the frequency of use of selected community-based services, individually and in the aggregate?
- How does the use of these services change over a 2-year period?
- What differences exist in service use and service users for residents of different housing arrangements, including recent movers to congregate facilities?

LITERATURE REVIEW

Most research on service use by older persons has adopted Andersen's (1968) behavioral model (Calsyn & Winter, 1999, 2000; Kosloski & Montgomery, 1994; Lynch, Harrington, & Newcomer, 1999; Mitchell & Krout, 1998; Wolinsky, 1994). Originally developed to illustrate the use of formal medical services, this framework has been applied to a broad array of social and health services used by older adults (Mitchell & Krout, 1998). Researchers applying the behavioral framework use either individual service-use measures or a summed service-use score. Researchers (Kosloski & Montgomery, 1994; Mitchell & Krout, 1998) have grouped services by type (e.g., health services) when applying this behavioral model.

The most common application of the behavioral model groups correlates of service use into predisposing, enabling, and need factors. Predisposing characteristics include demographics, social structure, and health beliefs. Enabling factors include personal or family and community resources. Need factors include real and perceived exigency, both medical and psychosocial. Need factors also include health problems and functional difficulties. Overall, previous research using this approach has shown that need factors tend to be the strongest correlates of service use and that the behavioral model is better suited to explaining social-service as opposed to medical-service utilization (Mitchell & Krout, 1998).

Space limitations preclude a review of what is known about the utilization of each community service, but it is useful to consider some generalizations concerning overall use and findings about several services that emerged as important in the *Pathways* study. One generalization is that the rate of service use varies with the service in question and is higher for elders with functional difficulties. Second, studies have shown that the most common service used nationwide is the senior center (Krout, Cutler, & Coward, 1990; Logan & Spitze, 1994). However, for elders with functional disabilities, home-based service usage (home-delivered meals and home care) is higher (Logan & Spitze, 1994; Short & Leon, 1990). Third, while findings vary from study to study, need and predisposing factors are generally more likely to be found to be correlates of service use than are enabling factors (Logan & Spitze, 1994; Mitchell & Krout, 1998).

Health and home health services bear particular mention. Medicare and the availability of additional private health insurance result in considerable use of health services (physician and hospitalization) by older adults in the United States. On average, people age 65 and over have contact with a physician or health care workers associated with a physician 11.4 times per year (U.S. Department of Health and Human Services, 1999). Those who are older, have more disabilities, have higher education levels and live in urban areas visit physicians most often (Coward, Duncan, & Freudenberger, 1994; Mutran & Ferraro, 1988; Saag et al., 1998; U.S. Department of Health and Human Services, 1999). The relationship between gender and physician visits is unclear. Earlier research by Wolinsky (1978) and Wan and Arling (1983) did not find a relationship between the two variables. More recent findings, however, suggest that women visit physicians more often than men (Mutran & Ferraro, 1988; Rivnyak, Wan, Stegall, Jacobes, & Li, 1989). Help from family members does not appear to be related to physician visits but does have a positive relationship with specialist visits (Mitchell, Mathews, & Griffin, 1997).

The use of health services delivered in the home (home care) increased significantly during the 1990s as Medicare coverage for these services expanded significantly. Hing (1994) reports that 80% of home care consumers use skilled nursing care, 50% use personal care, and less than 20% use other types of services (physical therapy, homemaker/companion services, social services, and occupational or vocational services). A profile of home care consumers is difficult to construct because discrepancies in home care definitions include medical and nonmedical services (Wacker, Roberto, & Piper, 1998). Despite the discrepancies, several findings emerge in the research on home care service use: home care use increases as consumers grow older (Altman & Walden, 1993) and physical disability increases (Grabbe, Demi, Whittington, Jones, & Branch, 1995); rural residents are less likely to use it than urban ones (Saag et al., 1998); and the relationship between home care use and family support yields conflicting results, with researchers reporting no relationship or that family assistance both complements and replaces professional home care (Chappel & Blandford, 1991; McAuley & Arling, 1984; Mitchell, Matthews & Griffin, 1997).

Several supportive social services are also of interest. We noted earlier that senior centers are the most frequently used nonmedical community-based service. Rates tend to vary by community (Krout, 1989) and national data for 1990 indicate that about 15% of older adults use senior centers at least once a year (Krout, Cutler, & Coward, 1990). Centers tend to be used most often by people who have less education (Miner, Logan, & Spitz, 1993; Sabin, 1993), fewer disabilities, and lower incomes and who live alone and are female (Krout et al., 1990). The older old are more likely to use senior centers than their younger counterparts, but attendance does tend to diminish after the age of 85 (Wacker, Roberto, & Piper, 1998). The decline may be due to increasing frailty, because most center participants are relatively healthy (Krout et al., 1990).

Finally, transportation services are important because of their role in helping older adults to live at home when they can no longer drive and in providing access to many other services in the community. Public transportation is one option for those who cannot own and operate a vehicle, or do not want to, or cannot afford to. Some public transportation is specially designed for people with disabilities. Public transportation is used primarily by older adults who are female, are urban residents, have mild to moderate disabilities, and have low incomes (Wacker et al., 1998). Unfortunately, public transportation fails to meet the needs of many older adults (Straight, 1997).

METHODS

SAMPLE

This research analyzes data collected during two waves of interviews from self-selected respondents living in congregate housing ($n = 243$), a random sample of older adults residing in their own homes in the greater community ($n = 346$), respondents on a waiting list to move into a new senior housing facility ($n = 57$), and a small group who moved to the new facility between interviews ($n = 37$). The analyses in this chapter combine the random sample and the participants on the waiting list, while keeping the movers as a separate group, bringing the total number of community-dwelling older adults to 403. The facility sample is broken into two groups, based on the richness of the services in the facility: service-rich, which is composed of 127 residents living in a CCRC; and service-poor, which is composed of 116 residents living in government-subsidized public housing ($n = 30$), and both urban and rural independent living senior apartments ($n = 86$).

SAMPLE CHARACTERISTICS

The average age of respondents is 76. However, there are differences in the ages of the residents of the various housing types. Movers are the oldest group, averaging 83 years. The community residents average 74 years, while those in service-rich senior housing average 80 years, and those in service-poor housing average 78 years. Overall, the movers and the residents of the service-poor senior housing have the highest number of activity limitations. Community residents have the most frequent contact with their children but the least frequent contact with their neighbors. Residents of the service-poor senior housing give lower health ratings (6.7 out of 10) than residents of other arrangements. Fewer of the service-poor residents (11%) and movers (35%) are married, whereas 64% of the community residents and 59% of the service-rich retirement community residents are married. Annual household income varies by residence as well, with 81% of the service-poor senior housing residents earning $20,000 a year or less. In contrast, 66% of the residents of the service-rich housing, and 24% of the community residents have annual incomes equal to or exceeding $75,000.

DEPENDENT VARIABLES

Dependent variables used in this analysis measure the utilization of individual health and social community-based services as well as the change in this use over 2 years. In both interviews, respondents were asked whether they and/or their spouse were currently using seven selected services: home health care, homemaker assistance, home delivered meals, senior center, information and referral, transportation, and legal assistance. Within the data set, each service is designated as a separate variable and the data coded *1* if the service is used and *0* if it is not. Summed service-use scores are calculated by summing the service variables for both sets of interviews. Respondents are also asked about the frequency of visits to doctors and specialists as well as the frequency, duration, and reasons for hospital and nursing-home stays

Within the study county there are versions of two of these services (transportation and information and referral) that bear more detailed explanation. In regard to transportation: for a small fee, seniors can be picked up at their homes and taken to just about any place they would like to go within the county—to doctors' offices, to the bank, or to the grocery store. Called Gadabout, this service is staffed by volunteer drivers and is more flexible than the public bus system. Respondents in our study report use of Gadabout along with public transportation systems.

In regard to the information and referral telephone service: callers receive a description of the requested service, an address and phone number, and the name of the primary contact person. Older residents may also contact the senior center and the county Office for the Aging for appropriate referrals when services are needed. Respondents in the *Pathways to Life Quality* study include both avenues in their responses about using the information and referral service.

INDEPENDENT VARIABLES

As indicated earlier, we use Andersen's model that categorizes independent variables as need, predisposing, and enabling. Need variables used in this research include perceived health, the number of illnesses, and the number of activities of daily living (ADLs) that a person is limited in performing. Predisposing characteristics are those that exist prior to the use of health services, such as health beliefs or biological characteristics. Predisposing variables used in this research include age, gender, and prior use of services, which may also affect the likelihood of an individual to use services subsequently. Factors that facilitate the use of services—such as transportation, insurance coverage, financial resources, and relationships with others—are enabling characteristics. Respondents rate their current health on a scale from 1 to 10, with 10 indicating the very best of health. Also included in the interviews are measures of health-based activity limitations, social integration (Cutrona & Russell, 1987), frequency of contact with children and neighbors, frequency/amounts of assistance given and received by friends and family (Koenig, Westlund, George, Hughes, & Blazer, 1993), and chronic health conditions.

FINDINGS

COMMUNITY-BASED SERVICE USE

Approximately half of the sample was using at least one service at the time of each interview. At the time of the first interview, 52% were using at least one service (W1), and at the time of the second interview, the figure was 51% (W2). The average number of services used at wave 1 was 1.7 (.91), and at wave 2, the average was 1.6 (.93). Table 7.1 shows the percentage of respondents using each service and highlights significant changes between the two interviews.

TABLE 7.1 *Pathways to Life Quality* Respondent-Reports of Community-based Service Use

	Wave 1	Wave 2	X^2
Home health care	13.4%	5.6%	5.48*
Home delivered meals	5.4%	5.1%	3.55
Homemaker	11.9%	18.5%	26.99***
Legal assistance	10.5%	10.6%	.01
Information and referral	5.9%	7.8%	3.40
Senior center	20.0%	20.1%	2.40
Transportation	20.6%	15.1%	76.01***

* $p < .05$; ** $p < .01$; *** $p < .001$.

The most frequently used services are transportation, the senior center, and homemaker assistance. Although the use of home health care and community-based transportation decreased and the use of the homemaker service increased, the percentage of the sample using services did not change over time. The overall rate of service use in the *Pathways* sample is higher than is generally reported in the literature for older adults and is likely to be explained by several factors. First, our sample includes a greater proportion of residents of congregate facilities than is found among older adults in general, and such living arrangements often have information and referral links to services. Second, about 20% of our sample lives in a CCRC, where services are included in the life care contracts, and residents have the means to purchase additional services (e.g., home health care) so they can stay in their current housing situation. Third, the county in which the study has been conducted has a relatively robust service network for older adults.

Table 7.1 also presents data on change in the use of specific services. Some of the change in the use of these services may be explained by the fact that respondents are 2 years older and have become somewhat frailer and less mobile. The increased use of homemaker and information-referral services and the decline in the use of transportation services seem consistent with this observation. On the other hand, increasing age might lead to a greater need for transportation services as individual driving abilities lessen. The decline in the use of home health services does not seem to fit this scenario. Perhaps respondents receiving these services at time 1 had recovered, and community-based services were no longer needed. On the other hand, the decline of home health service use could reflect systemic factors such as changes in home health care agency reimbursement practices by the federal government or private insurance carriers. Finally, the overall use rate of three of the services (home-delivered meals, legal assistance, and senior centers) did not change. This suggests that the interest in and need for them is more constant than it is for the other services and that their availability did not change.

DIFFERENCES BY LIVING ARRANGEMENT

Table 7.2 shows the percentage of respondents using each service at wave 1 and wave 2, in the various housing arrangements. It is difficult to summarize the results in Table 7.2 because they encompass multiple comparisons based on time and place. Overall, differences by housing are found at wave 1 and wave 2 in nearly all of the services, with the exception of information and referral at both times and of legal assistance at wave 1. The percentage of respondents using any one of the services varies by residence, with a range of one third to three quarters, depending on the time (W1 or W2) and location. This wide variation explains the overall use rate of 50%. Service use is much higher among residents of senior housing. This could be a selection effect in that people in these facilities are older, in poorer health, have greater service needs, and may have better access to community-based services.

TABLE 7.2 Community-based Service Use at Each Interview by Wave 2
Housing Arrangement

	Community	Service-rich	Service-poor	Movers	X^2
Home health					
W1	1.3%	59.5%	5.4%	7.7%	29.34***
W2	4.2%	3.2%	11.6%	7.7%	11.05**
Homemaker					
W1	7.8%	6.4%	23.2%	33.3%	41.84***
W2	13.2%	17.5%	30.4%	41.0%	31.31***
Meals					
W1	3.0%	.8%	15.2%	12.8%	36.11***
W2	3.5%	4.0%	14.3%	0.0%	23.88***
Transportation					
W1	6.8%	55.1%	32.1%	17.9%	21.26***
W2	6.0%	27.0%	32.1%	20.5%	66.57***
Senior center					
W1	20.1%	10.4%	25.9%	35.9%	15.70***
W2	22.4%	7.9%	25.0%	23.1%	14.76**
Legal assistance					
W1	9.3%	14.4%	9.8%	12.8%	2.94
W2	10.2%	17.5%	5.4%	7.7%	9.92*
Referral					
W1	5.5%	4.9%	8.9%	5.1%	2.20
W2	6.5%	7.1%	11.6%	12.8%	4.69
Any service used					
W1	36.7%	76.2%	72.3%	64.1%	84.45***
W2	33.3%	54.8%	68.8%	64.1%	27.08***

* $p < .05$; ** $p < .01$; *** $p < .001$.

Service-poor residents are more likely to utilize meals and transportation services, whereas movers are more likely to use homemaker services and senior centers. The greater use of services such as transportation and meals by service-poor residents may reflect their lower incomes and poorer health. Service-poor housing residents are also relatively high users of homemaker services, but not as high as movers who are older on average and thus perhaps even more likely to need such services. Movers, along with service-poor residents, are more likely to report using senior centers. These organizations generally are more likely to be utilized by low- and moderate-income individuals.

Residents of service-rich housing are more likely to use legal assistance at wave 2 and much more likely to use home health services at wave 1. Service-rich housing residents may use legal services more because they are more likely to have assets to protect (financial planning and taxes). They may also be more aware of and have more need for legal instruments such as wills, health care proxies, and living wills. Residents of the CCRC are required to sign a complicated life care contract and may seek legal advice in that regard. Service-poor housing residents, on the other hand, may seek legal assistance because they lack the resources to afford even the most basic legal work. Remember, some community-based services are available to persons age 60 and over, regardless of income.

We also observe some dramatic changes in service use over time for several services. For example, service-rich housing residents are much, much more likely to use home health and transportation services at wave 1, but use of the former drops to almost zero and use of the latter by half at wave 2. We speculate that the service-rich housing residents may have been using home health services to help with recovery from episodic health problems and to delay movement from independent to assisted living within the facility. By wave 2, individuals have either recovered and no longer need the service or have moved to a higher level of care within the CCRC, where needed services are provided on-site. Residents of the service-poor facility and the community see increased use of home health services over time, probably because they experience more health problems. Additionally, movers report significant declines in the use of meals, senior centers, and legal assistance, but an increase in the use of referral services. The drop to zero in the use of meals by movers is most likely explained by their relocation to a congregate facility that provides meals. This facility also has on-site recreation services and other staff (social workers), and that probably explains the decreased use of the senior center and the increased referral to other services. With the completion of their move by wave 2, legal services may also be less necessary.

SERVICE USERS VERSUS NON-SERVICE USERS

By selecting those who used any one of the services at either wave 1 or wave 2 and comparing them to those who did not use any services, we see that service users are older on average (average age at W2 is 78) than non-service users (average age at W2 is 74). Services are used predominantly by unmarried women who reside in congregate living environments. There are no differences in the types of chronic health conditions of those who use services compared to those who do not use services. These results are not presented in tabular form in this chapter.

CHARACTERISTICS OF SERVICE USERS

In order to test for differences among the service users in the various housing arrangements, ANOVA tests were run. *Service user* is defined as the use of any service at either W1 or W2. The percentage of service users in

TABLE 7.3 Difference in Profiles of Service Users in the Varied Living Arrangements

		SS	*df*	*MS*	*F*
Wave 1					
Summed use	Between	61.28	3	20.43	19.51***
	Within	468.94	448	1.05	
Health rating	Between	90.80	3	30.27	7.70***
	Within	1777.62	452	3.93	
Activity limitations	Between	289.54	3	96.51	15.31***
	Within	2855.51	453	6.30	
Children contacts	Between	1324.05	3	441.35	3.67**
	Within	5459.02	454	120.24	
Neighbor visits	Between	115.87	3	38.62	14.91***
	Within	1165.34	450	2.59	
Wave 2					
Age	Between	2218.51	3	739.51	14.23***
	Within	23643.85	455	51.97	
Summed use	Between	16.45	3	5.48	4.91**
	Within	507.39	454	1.12	
Health rating	Between	76.68	3	739.50	14.23***
	Within	1961.81	453	4.33	
Activity limitations	Between	295.65	3	98.55	11.54***
	Within	3885.57	455	8.54	
Hospital stays	Between	12.04	3	4.01	3.84**
	Within	190.37	182	1.05	
Children contacts	Between	4498.00	3	1499.33	13.55***
	Within	45032.01	407	1106.40	
Neighbor visits	Between	35281.16	3	11760.39	140.69***
	Within	37782.21	452	83.59	
Give help	Between	269.51	3	89.84	20.43***
	Within	2000.49	455	4.40	
Social integration	Between	2.11	3	.70	4.40**
	Within	72.56	453	.16	

* $p < .05$; ** $p < .01$; *** $p < .001$.

the various housing arrangements at W1 and W2 are shown in Table 7.3. Included in the ANOVA analyses are the total number of services used in W1 and W2, to test whether residents of the different living arrangements use more services than others; age; disability rates, activity limitations, health conditions, frequency of social contacts, and self-assessed health, all at W2.

In the first interview, differences in the total number of services used are seen in residents of service-rich and service-poor senior housing and community residents. Service-rich senior-housing residents received the most services, and community residents received the fewest.

At the time of the second interview, we see that the total number of services used was less for residents of service-rich senior housing compared to those in service-poor senior housing. The movers are significantly older (83) than either the service-rich (80) or the service-poor (79) senior-housing service users. The service users in the community sample are significantly younger (76) than those living in other arrangements. Community-service users have fewer activity limitations than those in service-poor housing and the movers, whereas the movers have significantly more limitations than do the service-using residents of the service-rich senior housing. Self-assessed health is similar for service users of each housing type and for the movers, although the community respondents rate their health higher than do those who live in service-poor senior housing. There are no differences in the number of physician visits or in the length of hospital stays, although service users in the service-poor senior housing had a greater number of hospital stays (2.0) than did community respondents (1.34).

Among service users, social integration scores are lower for the movers than for the service-using community respondents. Movers and residents of both service-rich and service-poor senior housing have contact with their neighbors more than community residents. Contact with children also varies among the groups, with the movers having contact with their children fewer days per year than community residents. Additionally, service-rich senior housing residents see their children less often than the community respondents and the residents of service-poor housing. There were no differences in the reported amount of assistance received from friends and family, but the amount of help given did differ, with community respondents providing significantly more than the other groups. However, service-rich senior housing residents provided more assistance than did the movers or the service-poor residents.

In sum, we see that service users differ based on their residential category. Those residing in service-rich senior housing show a decrease in their overall use of home-based services, particularly home health care. Movers to senior housing, were older than service users currently living in senior housing and they had more activity limitations than those in service-rich senior housing. Self-assessed health was similar for service users in all living environments. Community service users have less frequent contact with friends and neighbors, yet give more assistance to others than do residents of other arrangements. In the senior housing facilities, the more service-rich the residence, the less contact residents have with their children.

CHANGE AND STABILITY IN SERVICE USE

Overall service use does not change statistically when comparing the percentage of the sample that used any services, but there are changes in which individuals use each service. Table 7.4 shows that at a minimum, 80% of the individuals did not change their use or nonuse of the services we examined. Equal percentages stop and start using three of the seven services (home delivered meals, senior center, and legal services), with from 6 to 18% of the sample stopping or starting use, depending on the service used. This relatively stable pattern could reflect a variety of factors, including a stable level of program availability or overall constant levels of need and demand. Several services (home health care and transportation) show more people stopping than starting use. These services witness a decline in overall use by our sample that could have been caused by a variety of factors, such as less need or less availability of service. Home health care is often given for short periods of time as clients recover fairly quickly from acute

TABLE 7.4 Change in Use of Community-based Services

	Ceased using	No change	Began using
Home health	11.6	84.7	3.7
Homemaker	5.8	81.9	12.3
Home meals	3.1	93.9	3.0
Senior center	8.9	82.2	8.9
Transportation	13.2	82.1	4.7
Legal services	8.9	82.5	8.6
Referral service	4.6	88.8	6.6

Note: $n = 687$.

health problems or because health care payers such as Medicare and private insurers limit the number of visits and days of coverage. It is interesting that so few respondents indicate they began using home health care. On the other hand, a greater percentage of the sample started using homemaker services, while a larger percentage started using information and referral, compared to the percentage that ceased using the service.

Using ANOVA tests, differences are seen in the number of people starting and stopping each service by living arrangement in three of the seven services: home health care ($F = 137.67$; $df = 3, 668$; $p < .001$), transportation ($F = 44.86$; $df = 3,669$; $p < .001$), and home-delivered meals ($F = 4.66$; $df = 3, 667$; $p < .01$). Greater numbers of residents of the service-rich senior housing ceased using home health care and transportation. A greater proportion of those who moved between interviews stopped using home-delivered meals.

IMPLICATIONS FOR POLICY, PRACTICE, AND RESEARCH

The data reported in this chapter show that community-based service utilization varies considerably, depending on the service. This variation likely reflects a combination of factors, including need for the services, service availability and accessibility, and overall system capacity. We do not know how much unmet need for exists these services, but one could also view the data as indicating that the levels of service use are appropriate and that the service system is working as it should. One implication of the findings, then, is that the need for different types of services varies in this community (and others) and thus the resources devoted to various services should reflect this fact. Use of senior centers and transportation is more prevalent in the *Pathways* sample than is the use of home-delivered meals and information and referral. Higher levels of use can both increase costs and lead to savings because of the economies of scale. At the same time, some services are generally more expensive to deliver per unit of service than others, (e.g. home health care versus senior center programming), which can increase the total number of dollars needed for those services, even if prevalence of use is lower. These points also suggest a number of research questions about the relative importance of factors in explaining utilization levels of various services, including service accessibility, availability, and information; population characteristics; and the health and social needs of the older population.

Planning for service use over time is an ongoing challenge to service providers; another implication of the data is that considerable variability exists in the degree of this challenge, depending on the service. Home health and homemaker services show the largest changes in overall use over time, and this volatility can make planning for staffing and other resources more difficult. These services, in particular, would benefit from flexible and responsive program operation and priorities, staffing, and budgeting. Utilization of other services such as senior centers, home-delivered meals, and legal assistance remained unchanged overall, so one could argue that these services would face less difficulty in planning for resources over time, assuming that our sample reflects countywide use patterns.

The data also reveal that utilization patterns vary for individuals. The services experience client turnover ranging from 6% for home-delivered meals to 18% for homemaker services (adding together the percentages of the sample reporting beginning or ending each service). The amount of turnover has implications for service planning, delivery, and costs as services with higher turnover have to spend more time, relatively, on functions such as client intake, assessment, and integration into programs. What are the implications of high client turnover for staff training, program planning, and outcomes measurement? How do these impacts vary by service? These are important research questions.

Other implications of the data are the variations in service utilization for the different housing arrangements of the older adults in our sample. These differences can be attributed to many factors, including the needs of the people in that housing, the availability of on-site services, the accessibility and proximity to off-site services, and the fit between the available services and the needs of the residents. Assuming that use levels reflect service need, it is clear that such need varies considerably based on the type of housing arrangement. Based on our findings, managers of congregate housing should provide information about or links to certain kinds of services (or provide them on site) as opposed to others. Our findings also suggest that programs could be developed to decrease the conditions that lead to the need for service use. A fundamental research question here is the degree to which residents come to various housing situations with service needs as opposed to developing them over time as they age in place there. What programs can be put in place, particularly in congregate housing, to impact service needs over time?

Finally, findings concerning which individuals in the sample use services also have implications for service providers and housing managers. Service users tend to be unmarried women living in congregate residential settings. These women tend to have longer hospital stays, have less support, and have lower incomes, meaning that the government (Medicare and Medicaid) pays for the majority of the services received. Therefore, there may be limits on the amount or duration of home care, suggesting that if these older adults' needs are not met during the home care period, they stand a greater risk of relapse and subsequent rehospitalization. For older adults whose levels of health decline to the point where they require more intensive care that outside providers cannot meet, the likely solution would be relocation to a nursing home—a prospect that most older adults strongly dislike. This suggests a number of research questions. Would the expense of extended, long-term, home-based services and education programs following a hospital stay allow those older adults to remain in their current homes longer? Would it be less expensive than the daily cost of nursing home care? In government-subsidized public housing, is it beneficial to provide an on-site social worker to coordinate linkages to outside service agencies and assist in the oversight of care for their older residents? Would such an arrangement be of interest to housing managers, service providers, government housing agencies, and older adults residing in congregate housing?

SUMMARY AND CONCLUSIONS

This chapter examines changes in the use of community-based services by older adults over a 2-year period in a sample of 403 community dwellers compared to a convenience sample of 243 residents of congregate housing, of which 127 were residing in service-rich senior housing and 116 in service-poor senior housing. Our research shows that older adults have a need for and make use of a wide variety of community-based services. At each interview, approximately half of the sample were using at least one service. The prevalence of use varies considerably depending on the particular service, with use of senior centers and transportation reported by the largest percentage of the sample. Changes in use over a 2-year period are found for some services, whereas others show a relatively stable pattern of use. In addition, turnover in the percentage of the sample using a particular service also varies, but most individuals did not change their use or nonuse of a particular service.

Residential differences are found for most of the services. Service-poor housing residents use more home health care and home-delivered meals, whereas service-rich housing seniors use the senior center less often, and community residents use public transportation services less often. These differences reflect an undetermined combination of variation in the following factors: individual need by housing environment; service availability, both on site and in the community; and other factors, such as service access and knowledge. Across all of the residential types, we see an increase in the proportion of residents using homemaker assistance. We also find that service user characteristics vary by housing, with those in more service-rich environments having less frequent contact with their children and providing less assistance to others. Service-poor residents use more services and have more frequent hospital stays. Community dwelling residents are younger, use fewer services, and provide more informal support to family and friends. Movers are older, have more activity limitations, and have consistent rates of service use pre- and postmove.

These findings raise significant questions for researchers, practitioners, and housing planners and policy makers. What factors explain differences in service use by individuals, prevalence of use of specific services, changes in use of specific services, and variations in use patterns or different housing environments? What are the implications of variation in the prevalence of service use? What are the implications of variations in change of service use and users? How do these variations affect the service network collectively, and how do they affect the resources and planning of individual services? Do utilization patterns reflect the most appropriate and cost-effective use of service resources? How much need is not addressed by the existing services? How can services better identify at-risk residents so as to both target services and intervene at an earliest point, thereby promoting and prolonging health, well-being, and independence? Data from wave 3 of the *Pathways* study will provide additional insight into service-use patterns that will contribute to greater understanding of these questions and their solutions.

REFERENCES

Altman, B., & Walden, D. (1993). *Home health care: Use, expenditures, and sources of payment* (AHCPR Publication No. 93-0040: National Medical Expenditures Survey Research Findings No. 15). Rockville, MD: Public Health Service.

Andersen, R. M. (1968). *A behavioral model of families' use of health services* (Research Series No. 25). Chicago: University of Chicago, Center for Health Administration Studies.

Andersen, R. M. (1995). Revisiting the behavioral model and access to medical care: Does it matter? *Journal of Health and Social Behavior, 36*(1), 1–10.

Bassuk, K. (1999). NORC supportive service programs: Effective and innovative programs that support seniors living in the community. *Care Management Journals, 1*(2), 132–137.

Beigel, D. E., Farkas, K. J., & Wadsworth, N. (1994). Social service programs for older adults and their families. In P. K. H. Kim (Ed.), *Services to the aging and aged: Public policies and programs.* New York: Garland.

Calsyn, R. J., & Winter, J. P. (1999). Who attends senior centers? *Journal of Social Service Research, 26*(2), 53–69.

Calsyn, R. J., & Winter, J. P. (2000). Predicting different types of service use by the elderly: The strength of the behavioral model and the value of interaction terms. *Journal of Applied Gerontology, 19*(3), 284–303.

Chappell, N., & Blandford, A. (1991). Informal and formal care: Exploring the complementarity. *Ageing and Society, 11*(3), 299–317.

Coward, R. T., Duncan, R. P., & Freudenberger, K. M. (1994). Residential differences in the use of formal services prior to entering a nursing home. *The Gerontologist, 24*(1), 44–49.

Cutrona, C. E., & Russell, D. W. (1987). The provisions of social relationships and adaptation to stress. *Advances in Personal Relationships, 1,* 37–67.

Grabbe, L., Demi, A. S., Whittington, F., Jones, J. M., & Branch, L. G. (1995). Functional status and the use of formal home care in the year before death. *Journal of Aging and Health, 7*(3), 339–364.

Hing, E. (1994). *Characteristics of elderly home health patients: Preliminary data from the 1992 national home and hospice care survey* (Advance Data from Vital and Health Statistics, No. 247). Hyattsville, MD: National Center for Health Statistics.

Kassner, E., & Bectel, R. W. (1998). *Midlife and older Americans with disabilities: Who gets help?* Washington, DC: AARP.

Kim, P. K. H. (Ed.). (1994). *Services to the aging and aged: Public policies and programs.* New York: Garland.

Koenig, H. G., Westlund, R. E., George, L. K., Hughes, D. C., & Blazer, D. G. (1993). Abbreviating the Duke Social Support Index for use in chronically ill elderly individuals. *Psychosomatics, 34,* 61–69.

Kosloski, K., & Montgomery, R. J. V. (1994). Investigating patterns of service use by families providing care for dependent elders. *Journal of Aging and Health, 6*(1), 17–37.

Krout, J. A. (1989). *Senior Centers in America.* Westport, CT: Greenwood.

Krout, J. A., Cutler, S. J., & Coward, R. T. (1990). Correlates of senior center participation: A national analysis. *The Gerontologist, 30*(1), 72–79.

Logan, J. R., & Spitze, G. (1994). Informal support and the use of formal services by older Americans. *Journals of Gerontology: Social Sciences, 49*(1), S25–S34.

Lynch, M., Harrington, C., & Newcomer, R. (1999). Predictors of use of chronic care services by impaired members in the social health maintenance organization demonstration. *The Journal of Applied Gerontology, 18*(3), 283–304.

McAuley, W. J., & Arling, G. (1984). Use of in-home care by very old people. *Journal of Health and Social Behavior, 25*(1), 54–64.

Miner, S., Logan, J. R., & Spitz, G. (1993). Predicting the frequency of senior center attendance. *The Gerontologist, 33*(5), 650–657.

Mitchell, J., & Krout, J. A. (1998). Discretion and service use among older adults: The behavioral model revisited. *The Gerontologist, 38*(2), 159–168.

Mitchell, J., Mathews, H. F., & Griffin, L. W. (1997). Health and community based service use: Differences between elderly African Americans and whites. *Research on Aging, 19*(2), 199–122.

Mutran, E., & Ferraro, K. R. (1988). Medical need and use of services among older men and women. *Journal of Gerontology, 43*(5), S162–S171.

Rivnyak, M. H., Wan, T. T. H., Stegall, M. H., Jacobes, M., & Li, S. (1989). Ambulatory care use among the noninstitutionalized elderly. *Research on Aging, 11*(3), 292–311.

Saag, K. G., Doebbeling, B. N., Rohrer, J. E., Kolluri, S., Peterson, R., Hermann, M. E., & Wallace, R. B. (1998). Variation in tertiary prevention and health service utilization among the elderly: The role of urban-rural residence and supplemental insurance. *Medical Care, 36*(7), 965–976.

Sabin, E. P. (1993). Social relationships and mortality among the elderly. *Journal of Applied Gerontology, 12*(1), 44–60.

Short, P., & Leon, P. (1990). *Use of home and community services by persons age 65 and older with functional difficulties* (DHHS Publication No. PHS 90-3466). Rockville, MD: U.S. Public Health Service.

Straight, A. (1997). *Community transportation survey.* Washington, DC: AARP.

U.S. Department of Health and Human Services. (1999). *Health, United States, 1999, with Health and Aging Chartbook* (DHHS Publication No. PHS 99–1232). Washington, DC: U.S. Government Printing Office.

Wacker, R. R., Roberto, K. A., & Piper, L. W. (1998). *Community resources for older adults: Programs and services in an era of change.* Thousand Oaks, CA: Pine Forge.

Wan, T. T., & Arling, G. (1983). Differential use of health services among functionally disabled elders. *Research on Aging, 5,* 411–431.

Whitelach, C. J., & Noelker, L. S. (1996). Caregiving and caring. In James E. Birren (Ed.) *Encyclopedia of Gerontology: Age, Aging and the Aged* (pp. 253–268). San Diego: Academic.

Wolinsky, F. D. (1978). Assessing the effects of predisposing, enabling, and illness-morbidity characteristics on health service utilization. *Journal of Health and Social Behavior, 19,* 384–396.

Wolinsky, F. D. (1994). Health services utilization among older adults: Conceptual, measurement, and modeling issues in secondary analysis. *The Gerontologist, 34*(4), 470–475.

SECTION 5

Well-Being and Adjustment

CHAPTER 8

Residential Differences in Life Stress and Perceived Health

Elaine Wethington

T he extensive research literature on life events and other stressors documents a relationship between stressor exposure and increased psychological distress (e.g., Pearlin, Liberman, Menaghan, & Mullan, 1981) and decreased physical health (Holmes & Rahe, 1967). These effects have been replicated in studies of older people (e.g., Glass, Kasl, & Berkman, 1997).

Very little is known about the relationship between stressors and residential settings in older people. Previous chapters in this volume suggest that the relationship is bidirectional. Declining health, increasing physical disability, and widowhood are often cited as reasons for relocating to senior housing facilities, especially to those offering assistance for the activities of daily living (see chapter 6). It is also possible, however, that different types of residential settings provide relief from or protection from some types of stressors. They may do this by providing a safe, controlled environment, providing housekeeping and meals, and increasing opportunities for social interaction (see chapters 4 and 5 of this volume).

This chapter examines the distribution of and exposure to life events and chronic stressors in the *Pathways to Life Quality* study. It examines the distribution of those events in tandem with residential and relocation status. It relates the occurrence of life stressors to changes in perceived physical health status and in personal mastery of life. This chapter accounts for other personal factors contributing to perceived physical health and mastery, such as cognitive difficulties, previous health status, and social integration. Declines in the perceived sense of control over areas of life that are salient to identity have been associated with increased mortality among older people (Krause, 2000).

The chapter addresses several specific questions. First, does exposure to events differ by relocation and by residential setting? If so, can these differences be explained by aging per se, by declines in health that may lead to relocation to housing that offers assisted living (see chapter 2, this volume), or by other losses that are associated with aging, such as the death of family members? Second, do life events and, more importantly, chronic stressors that may have accumulated over the life course reduce perceived physical health and personal mastery among older people? Third, do more protected residential settings mitigate the negative impacts of stressors on physical health and the sense of mastery?

AGING, STRESSORS, AND HEALTH

This chapter applies a variant of the selective optimization and compensation perspective (Smith & Baltes, 1997) to explore the relationship between health and exposure to stressors. The selective optimization and compensation (SOC) perspective predicts that losses increase in number as people age. It also predicts that as people age, their resources to compensate for losses can decline. Generally, people selectively optimize those areas of life in which they can exert some control over outcomes. However, cognitive declines and social isolation constrain and limit individual adaptation (Smith & Baltes, 1997). Thus, emotional adjustment to losses in later adulthood will be more difficult for those who are having greater difficulty maintaining social relationships and, more generally, for those with lower levels of preexisting social integration and support (LeFrancois, Leclerc, Hamel, & Gaulin, 2000).

Although the relationship between life stressors and perceived physical and mental health have been addressed in other longitudinal studies (e.g., Haug, Belgrave, & Gratton, 1984), few studies have examined the association in the context of housing selection and choice. Promoters of congregate housing for older people offer social activities as an important attraction, particularly for those adults who find it increasingly difficult to maintain physical independence. Indeed, social activities are believed to be a major factor in maintaining productivity and health among older people (Rowe & Kahn, 1998). Yet the very fact that congregate housing offers services to those whose health is less than optimal encourages those who are more frail and unhealthy to live in settings that may expose them to more events involving loss, such as deaths of friends and acquaintances.

There is also a possible "contagion" effect of witnessing infirmity and illness as others of the same age decline.

Senior residences also vary in the services they offer and, thus, the protection they provide from the strains of daily living. The senior facilities in the *Pathways to Life Quality* study offer a wide variety of services, all the way from life care at the continuing care retirement community (CCRC) to minimal assistance for daily living at service-poor residential settings (see chapter 2). On average, the members of the *Pathways* sample with the lowest incomes and the fewest accumulated assets were already residents of service-poor facilities when the study began. This means that the residents of the service-poor facilities had likely experienced a larger number of stressors, as well as poorer health across their lives (see chapter 6). Thus, another possible reason that older people may not show benefits from relocating to congregate housing may be the social, economic, and health selection factors that bring them into senior housing.

Health and sensory factors associated with aging may also limit the positive aspects of congregate housing. Increasing health problems and sensory decline limit social participation and can make normal social interaction difficult. Cognitive decline may bring about interpersonal difficulties and isolation, reducing available resources for coping when life events and chronic stressors occur (Cervilla & Prince, 1997; Ormel, Oldenhinkel, & Brilman, 2001) and limiting resilience in well-being (Smith & Baltes, 1997). On the other hand, the SOC perspective also implies that the continued ability to select a supportive setting in which one can optimize personal and social resources may lead to better maintained physical health over a longer term (Schultz & Heckhausen, 1996). The SOC perspective also implies a different direction in the relationship between residential setting and events involving loss—specifically, that events that threaten continued physical health will encourage relocation to a more supportive housing arrangement.

Social and personal resources, such as social integration, optimal role participation, and mastery, may moderate the impact of stressful events (Wheaton, 1999). (See also chapters 4 and 5 of this volume.) More specifically, Murrell and Norris (1991) described four different approaches— differential exposure, resource deterrent, differential vulnerability, and social buffering—to understanding how social and personal resources and contexts may moderate or exacerbate the stressful impact of events on older people. These four approaches suggest ways in which residential settings can have an impact on health, as well as on the selection factors that guide people to particular settings. In addition, these four approaches are quite compatible with the SOC perspective, although they place somewhat more emphasis on support from the social context than on personality resources.

First, the differential exposure hypothesis predicts that people with fewer economic resources are exposed to more stressors, both currently and cumulatively over time. This perspective predicts that those older people who reside in service-poor settings (see chapter 2) may experience more events and chronic stressors. Second, the resource deterrent hypothesis asserts that in lower resource settings, social support is less available to help people cope with the impacts of stressors. This perspective implies that those in service-poor residential settings will have lower levels of support. Third, the differential vulnerability hypothesis posits that stressors have greater impacts on those who are personally or socially more vulnerable, such as residents of service-poor settings (see chapter 6 of this volume). Fourth, the social buffering hypothesis implies that the impacts of stressors are moderated by the availability of social support. Where greater assistance to support daily living is available, the impacts of stressors may be moderated.

The ability of control, or mastery, to buffer the effects of stress is also well known (e.g., Lazarus & Folkman, 1984; Pearlin et al., 1981). In general, the belief that one can master and control the environment is associated with perceiving threats to be less stressful (Lazarus & Folkman, 1984). A higher sense of mastery is associated with more effective management of stressors (Pearlin & Schooler, 1978). However, the sense of personal mastery tends to erode when there is an accumulation of chronic stressors that cannot be mitigated by individual action (Pearlin et al., 1981). Research on mastery thus suggests that those who move to senior housing facilities may experience a decaying sense of mastery over time, particularly when relocation is accompanied by accumulating health problems.

These varying perspectives on the relationship between stressor exposure and perceived physical health imply a number of hypotheses about the distribution and impact of life stressors among older people in the *Pathways* sample who reside in various residential settings:

• Hypothesis 1: Residential setting will be related to the number of life events and chronic stressors experienced in the recent past. Specifically,
  (a) older people living in service-poor facilities will report more chronic stressors;
  (b) older people living in any senior facility (including service-rich

facilities) will have experienced more health-related events and stressors in the past 2 years.

- Hypothesis 2: Recent movers to senior-housing facilities will have experienced more recent health events and increases in functional limitations.
- Hypothesis 3: People living in senior facilities will report lower perceived health and lower perceived mastery over life than older people living in the community.
- Hypothesis 4: Older people experiencing more frequent health events, life events, chronic stressors, cognitive problems, and increases in functional limitations will experience a decline in perceived health over time.
- Hypothesis 5: Declines in perceived health as a consequence of life stressors will be exacerbated among those with preexisting lower levels of perceived social integration and personal mastery.
- Hypothesis 6: People experiencing more frequent health events, life events, chronic stressors, cognitive problems, and increases in functional limitations will experience a decline in personal mastery over time.

METHODS

SAMPLE

The analyses presented in this chapter are conducted using data from wave 1 and wave 2 in the *Pathways* longitudinal sample. The analyses exclude community volunteers and spouses of primary respondents as well as respondents under the age of 60. The maximum number of participants for these analyses is 616; however, missing data reduce the effective number to 551 or to 562 in multivariate analyses (depending on the choice of dependent variable). In this analysis sample, 56% live in community housing at wave 2; 23% live in service-rich facilities (the CCRC and two facilities that provide assisted-living services); and 21% live in service-poor facilities (see chapter 1 of this volume for a more complete description of facilities). In the past 2 years, 26 respondents have moved to service-rich facilities; 4 have moved to service-poor facilities.

MEASURES OF PERCEIVED PHYSICAL HEALTH AND PERSONAL MASTERY

Physical Health

The major dependent variables are perceived physical health at wave 2. Two 1-item measures are used. The first, Comparative Perceived Health, is the question In general, how would you say your health is, compared to other people your age? Would you say excellent, good, fair, or poor? The item is scored so that the high score of 4 represents excellent health. The mean score at wave 2 is 3.15 (SD = .75). This and similarly worded questions are used extensively in studies of physical health and the item relates well to states of physical disability, illness, and even mortality (Centers for Disease Control and Prevention, 2000; Idler & Benyamini, 1997). It is included in these analyses because it enables comparison to other studies of older people that have used this question. The second measure of health used is the Perceived Health Ladder, used as well in chapter 6 of this volume. The wording of this question is How would you describe your health these days, where 0 is poor health and 10 is the very best health? At wave 2, the mean level is 7.36 (SD = 2.10).

Personal Mastery

The measure of personal mastery used in this chapter is the Mastery scale, a seven-item scale developed by Pearlin and associates (Pearlin & Schooler, 1978). The measure is widely used. The sample mean is 2.96 at wave 2 (SD = .40).

MEASURES OF STRESSOR EXPOSURE AND SOCIAL AND PERSONAL RESOURCES

Life Events

Life events were assessed at wave 2. The recall period for events is the previous 2 years (that is, since the wave 1 interview). Two types of events were assessed: personal health events and other life events (primarily losses and threats of loss).

Three types of personal health events are summed to form an index of health events: new diagnosis of an illness, recent worsening of a preexisting personal illness, and hospitalization. The number of health events ranges from 0 to 3, with a mean of .73 (SD = .90).

A sum of other life events is also constructed. The index includes divorce, separation, legal problems, death of a close family member, deaths of other family members and friends (up to four were recorded), recent illness of a spouse, recent hospitalization of a spouse, and new diagnosis of a family member's illness. The average number of other life events reported is 1.49 (SD = 1.36), with a range of 0 to 7.

Although not a comprehensive list of possible life events (for example, recent financial events are not assessed), the interview adequately represents the types of events believed to increase as people age, become sick, and die (for comparison, see Glass, Kasl, & Berkman, 1997; Ormel, Oldenhinkel, & Brilman, 2001).

A possible limitation of this measure of life events is that it consists entirely of discrete events, excluding chronic stressors. Chronic stressor exposure is assessed using separate measures described below. With sufficient additional data (not currently available for the *Pathways* study), the measure of life events exposure could be made more sensitive by weighting for level of threat or severity and by taking account of the nature of new illnesses (whether life-threatening or disabling) and the degree of closeness to friends and family who have become ill or died.

Chronic Stressors

Researchers are increasingly calling for the inclusion of chronic stressors in the routine assessment of exposure to life stressors (e.g., Wethington, Almeida, Brown, Frank, & Kessler, 2001; Wheaton, 1999). For example, Lepore, Miles, & Levy (1997) demonstrated that chronic stressors are more closely related to increases in psychological distress than are life events. Although the assessment of chronic stressors in the *Pathways* study was not designed to be comprehensive, it does include a number of measures of chronic stressor exposure typically associated with higher rates of psychological and physical distress. These measures include providing care to another person on a daily basis (Aneshensel, Pearlin, Mullan, Zarit, & Whitlach, 1995), living in small or crowded housing (Evans, Wells, Chan, & Saltzman, 2001), frequent marital conflict (Lepore, 1995), and serious financial problems (Pearlin & Schooler, 1978). The chronic stressor index is constructed as a rational scale, assigning one point to each situation that met a preestablished criterion of severity (e.g., marital conflict at least weekly, not having enough money to meet needs). The mean number of chronic stressors is .26 ($SD = .50$), with a sample range of 0 to 3.

In order to measure the impact of chronic stressors in a way that parallels life events, chronic stressors involving health were assessed in a separate measure. Chronic stressors involving health were assessed using an indicator of increase in functional limitations between waves 1 and 2. The index is coded 1 if there was an increase of at least two functional limitations from those reported at wave 1. In the analysis sample, 19.5% report an increase in functional limitations.

Cognitive Problems

The *Pathways* study does not include a standard assessment tool of cognitive difficulties. The study protocol involved screening potential participants for cognitive problems by speaking with family and household members about whether the older resident in the household would be able to do the interview. Thus potential subjects who had difficulties with maintaining conversation and with memory were excluded as ineligible. However, after each interview, interviewers evaluated the quality of the interaction, rating the difficulty the respondent had in remembering things, as well as attention span and memory. These three interviewer observations were averaged to form a score of Cognitive Problems. The mean of this index is 1.23 ($SD = .41$), with an alpha reliability of .79. The wave 1 measure of cognitive problems is used in these analyses in order to avoid confounding with the wave 2 measures used as outcomes. Although by no means a standard measure of cognitive decline, the wave 1 measure of cognitive problems is associated with lower scores on the wave 1 perceived physical health ladder ($r = -.199$, $p < .001$) and the wave 1 comparative perceived health item ($r = -.144$, $p < .001$). It is also associated with sample attrition at wave 2 ($r = .167$, $p < .001$).

Social Resources

The Perceived Social Integration subscale from the Social Provisions Scale is used in these analyses as a measure of social support (Cutrona, Russell, & Rose, 1986). The scale is described fully in chapter 5 of this volume. The wave 1 measure of perceived social integration is used in these analyses because it preserves the most cases for longitudinal analyses. (Other Social Provisions subscales are not available from the CCRC founders at wave 1.) Also, the wave 1 social integration subscale is as strongly correlated with perceived health and personal mastery as the other subscales of the Social Provisions measure. The average level of perceived social integration is 3.21 ($SD = .44$). Married or partnered status at wave 2 (1 = married or partnered, 0 = not married) is also included as an indicator of social resources.

Personal Resources

The wave 1 measure of personal mastery (Pearlin & Schooler, 1978) is used as a measure of preexisting levels of mastery. The mean at wave 1 is 2.93 ($SD = .43$).

ANALYSIS STRATEGY

The analyses consist of four steps. First, the distributions of life events and chronic stressors at wave 2 are examined by residential setting and recent relocation. Second, levels of perceived health and personal mastery are assessed by residential setting and recent relocation. Third, stressor exposure (health events, other life events, and chronic stressors) is regressed at wave 2 on age, education, gender, residential setting, recent relocation, and personal and social resources at wave 1, including wave 1 perceived health, mastery, and cognitive problems. Finally, perceived health and personal mastery are regressed at wave 2 on all four types of stressor exposure, on the wave 1 measure of the outcome, and on the other predictors. This final analysis estimates how much stressor exposure and residential factors may account for changes in perceived health and personal mastery over time.

FINDINGS

RESIDENTIAL SETTINGS AND EXPOSURE TO STRESSORS

Contrary to expectations derived from the resource deterrence perspective, residents of service-poor facilities at wave 2 do not report significantly more health events or other life events than do other members of the sample (Table 8.1). Residents of the CCRC report significantly more recent health events than those who live in community housing. (No other group differences are significant.) People who live in the community report more other life events than those who live in facilities, even though facility residents are on average older than community residents. It is likely that community residents are, on average, more engaged in life and have larger social networks, thus leading to more frequent event exposure.

Residents of service-poor facilities report the greatest exposure to chronic stressors ($M = .43$). This is most likely to be the result of living in smaller apartments, being more involved in daily caregiving, and having a higher rate of financial problems. Residents of the complexes offering assisted living, although living in a service-rich environment, are the second most likely to experience chronic stressors. This is probably because the units feel too small in comparison to the residents' previous homes and because they are involved more frequently in daily caregiving. Residents of all of the senior facilities are more likely to report an increase in functional limitations since wave 1, in comparison to those who have lived continuously in the community.

TABLE 8.1 Percent Experiencing Life Events and Chronic Stressors in the Past 2 years, by Residential Setting at Wave 2

	CCRC	Assisted-living facilities	Service-poor facilities	Community housing	F ratio
Health events (mean)	.969	.800	.819	.615	4.95**
New personal illness onset	40 (41.7%)	14 (31.1%)	50 (39.4%)	125 (35.9%)	
Hospitalization	47 (48.9%)	18 (40.0%)	50 (39.4%)	83 (23.9%)	
Worsening personal illness	22 (22.9%)	17 (37.8%)	43 (33.9%)	77 (22.1%)	
Other life events (mean)	1.427	1.356	1.425	1.569	.691
Divorced or separated	5 (5.2%)	0 (0.0%)	7 (5.5%)	12 (3.4%)	
Death of close family member	22 (22.9%)	17 (37.8%)	44 (34.6%)	95 (27.3%)	
Death of another family member or close friend	36 (37.5%)	16 (35.6%)	50 (39.4%)	132 (37.9%)	
Onset of new illness in family	27 (28.1%)	19 (42.2%)	54 (42.5%)	103 (29.6%)	
Legal problems	5 (5.2%)	2 (4.4%)	4 (3.1%)	16 (4.6%)	
Onset of spouse illness[a]	11 (11.5%)	1 (2.2%)	1 (0.8%)	49 (14.1%)	
Spouse hospitalization[a]	16 (16.7%)	2 (4.4%)	2 (1.6%)	45 (12.9%)	
Chronic stressors (mean)	.208	.378	.425	.184	9.10***
Housing too small	15 (15.6%)	11 (24.4%)	37 (29.1%)	22 (6.3%)	
Daily caregiving	4 (4.2%)	6 (13.3%)	12 (9.4%)	30 (8.6%)	
Frequent marital conflicts	1 (1.0%)	0 (0.0%)	0 (0.0%)	4 (1.1%)	
Serious financial problems	0 (0.0%)	0 (0.0%)	5 (3.9%)	8 (2.3%)	
Increase in limitations (%)	32.1	30.0	30.2	15.1	6.90**
(n)	(96)	(45)	(127)	(348)	

[a]The percentages are calculated using the total subgroup n, rather than married respondents only.

*** $p < .001$; ** $p < .01$; * $p < .05$.

RELOCATION AND EXPOSURE TO STRESSORS

Those who have recently relocated to facilities ($N = 30$) do not report significantly more health events or other life events (not shown). However, they do report significantly more chronic stressors ($M = .43, p < .05$) and are marginally ($M = .33, p < .10$) more likely to report increased functional limitations than those who have not moved since wave 1.

RESIDENTIAL SETTING, PERCEIVED HEALTH, AND PERSONAL MASTERY

People who live in community housing at wave 2 consistently report higher perceived health and personal mastery (Table 8.2, panel 1). Among residents of senior housing, only residents of service-poor facilities differ significantly from community residents in perceived health and mastery. Recent movers to facilities (Table 8.2, panel 2) do not report worse perceived health than do those who have not moved (or community residents), but they do report significantly lower personal mastery. Both of these sets of findings might be explained by age; those who have recently relocated to facilities are significantly older (81.4 years) than the nonrelocating residents in the *Pathways* sample. Table 8.2, panel 3, explores that possibility by presenting the mean levels of perceived health and mastery by three age groups—60 to 69, 70 to 79, and 80 and older. Perceived health does not differ significantly by decade age groups, whereas personal mastery declines.

EXPOSURE TO STRESSORS AND PERCEIVED HEALTH

Table 8.3 presents a series of six regressions. The first three columns present regressions of health events, other events, and chronic stressors on demographic factors, residential setting, recent relocation, and preexisting perceived health, social integration, and personal mastery on three measures of life stressors, health events, other life events, and chronic stressors. Community residence at wave 2 is the excluded residential category. These three regressions confirm findings previously described but have the additional virtue of controlling for potentially confounding variables that might explain the relationship between residential setting and exposure to stressors. It is important to note that older people living in the CCRC at wave 2 are significantly more likely to report health events than are those living in the community at wave 2 ($b = .230, p < .05$), controlling for the potential confounders of age and preexisting health, both of which are also significantly related to reporting more health events (see Table 8.3, column 1). Exposure to other life events does not significantly differ by residential setting (see Table 8.3,

TABLE 8.2 Perceived Health and Mastery by Residential Setting, Relocation, and Age

	Comparative perceived health, W2	Perceived health ladder, W2	Personal mastery, W2
Residential setting			
CCRC	3.22	7.16	2.97
Assisted living	3.16	7.19	2.77
Service-poor facilities	2.84	6.56	2.81
Community housing	3.23***	7.32***	3.01***
Recent movers to facilities	3.13	7.07	2.79**[a]
Age group			
60–69	3.11	7.35	3.09
70–79	3.14	7.39	2.99
80–101	3.13	7.14	2.80***

*** $p < .001$; ** $p < .01$; * $p < .05$.
[a] Significantly lower than sample members who did not relocate to facilities.
W2, wave 2.

column 2). Exposure to chronic stressors is significantly higher in those who live in service-poor facilities ($b = .248$, $p < .001$) than in those who live in the community (see Table 8.3, column 3).

Columns 4 and 5 of Table 8.3 summarize the regressions of perceived physical health on age, gender, residential setting, recent relocation, and stressor exposure. The controls also include cognitive problems at wave 1, perceived social integration and mastery at wave 1, and perceived physical health at wave 1. The inclusion of wave 1 perceived physical health as a predictor transforms the two regressions into analyses of change in perceived physical health. The coefficients are interpreted as being tests of whether the levels of the predictors are associated with a significant change in perceived physical health over time. Cognitive problems, mastery, and perceived social integration at wave 1 are included to test whether they are associated with changes in perceived physical health. That is, they test whether they predict the trajectory of perceived health over and above the contribution of residential setting and stressor exposure.

People who live in service-poor facilities are significantly more likely to show a decline in comparative perceived health over time ($b = -.173$, $p < .05$), controlling for wave 1 perceived health and exposure to stressors.

TABLE 8.3 Regression of Wave 2 Life Stressors, Perceived Health and Mastery on Demographic Factors, Residential Setting, Social and Personal Resources, and Other Life Circumstances

	Health Events	Other Events	Chronic stressors	Comparative perceived health, W2	Perceived health ladder, W2	personal mastery, W2
	b	b	b	b	b	b
Age	.015**	-.006	-.008**	.011**	.028**	-.007***
Education	-.014	-.023	.031	.010	-.157	.036+
Female	.039	-.030	-.063	.088	.208	-.084**
Lives in CCRC	.230*	-.038	.056	-.016	-.175	-.074+
Assisted living	.330	-.617	.213	-.111	1.140+	-.075
Lives in service-poor facility	-.017	-.006	.248***	-.173*	-.258	-.089*
Recently moved to facility	-.375	.653	.057	.064	-1.150*	.050
Married/partnered, W2	.029	.433**	.021	.053	.172	-.080*
Cognitive problems, W1	.178+	-.001	-.012	.103	.084	-.008
Perceived health, W1[a]	-.191***	-.183**	-.053+	.473***	.505***	.016
Personal mastery, W1	.116	-.268	-.122*	.290***	.418*	.430***
Perceived social integration, W1	-.111	.294+	-.064	-.032	.034	.059+
Health events				-.140**	-.549***	-.019
Other life events				-.002	-.027	-.004
Chronic stressors				-.023	-.069	-.059*
Increase in limitations, W1–W2				-.174***	-.728***	-.082*
Intercept	-.027	2.30**	1.50***	-.073	.830	2.11***
F ratio	3.74***	2.41**	4.27***	20.74***	23.46***	23.22***
R²	.07	.05	.08	.38	.41	.41
R² (adjusted)	.05	.03	.07	.36	.39	.39
(n)	(562)	(562)	(562)	(551)	(557)	(555)

a In column 5, measured as Perceived health ladder, W1.
*** p < .001; ** p < .01; * p < .05; + p < .10.

A number of health events and an increase in functional limitations are associated with a significant decrease in the level of comparative perceived physical health over time, whereas other life events and chronic stressors are not associated with declines in perceived health. Higher mastery at wave 1 is associated with a significant increase in comparative perceived physical health. Age is significantly associated with an increase in comparative perceived health, possibly indicating a survivor effect.

The analysis of the perceived health ladder, which does not include the comparative frame, gives a somewhat different picture. Living in one of the two facilities that offer more extensive assisted-living services is associated with marginally higher perceived health in comparison to older members of the sample who are living in the community ($b = 1.197$, $p < .10$), whereas having recently moved into a facility is associated with significantly lower perceived health ($b = -1.193$, $p < .05$). As with comparative perceived health, age is significantly related to increases in perceived health, on average, as is wave 1 mastery. Health events and increases in functional limitations are significantly associated with declines in health, but other life events and chronic stressors are not.

EXPOSURE TO STRESSORS, SOCIAL AND PERSONAL RESOURCES, AND PERCEIVED HEALTH

Theories about the ways in which life events have an impact on perceived health assert, however, that psychosocial resources may moderate the impact of life events on perceived health. House, Umberson, and Landis (1988) suggested that preexisting levels of social integration (including marital or partner status) may moderate the impact of life events on health. Smith and Baltes (1997) asserted that declining cognitive faculties are associated with a general deterioration in well-being.

In order to evaluate the predictions of these perspectives, I reestimated the equations in columns 4 and 5 of Table 8.3, controlling for a series of interactions. The interactions were the products of the number of health events, other life events, and chronic stressors and (a) being married or partnered, (b) experiencing cognitive problems at wave 1, (c) perceived social integration at wave 1, and (d) personal mastery at wave 1. Because of multicollinearity among the interaction terms, each was entered in a separate equation. Of the 12 interactions tested, none were significant. In the *Pathways* sample, preexisting social and personal resources do not buffer the impact of stressor exposure on perceived health.

EXPOSURE TO STRESSORS AND PERSONAL MASTERY

The regression of perceived mastery on life stressors is presented in column 6 of Table 8.3. Living in the CCRC is associated with a marginal decrease in mastery ($b = -.076, p < .10$) in comparison to living in the community, and residing in a service-poor facility is associated with a significant decrease in mastery ($b = -.096, p < .05$). Among the measures of stressor exposure, chronic stressors and increase in functional limitations are associated with a significant decrease in mastery. Increasing age, being female, and being married are associated with decreasing mastery, while higher education is associated with increasing mastery over time.

IMPLICATIONS FOR RESEARCH, POLICY, AND PRACTICE

This chapter addressed several specific questions about the relationship between stressor exposure and perceived health and personal mastery across residential settings. First, does exposure to events differ by relocation and by residential setting? Second, do recent life events and, more important, chronic stressors that may have accumulated in later life, reduce perceived physical health and personal mastery among older people? Third, do more protected residential settings mitigate the negative impacts of stressors on physical health and the sense of mastery?

The findings show that residential setting is related to exposure to life stressors at wave 2. Overall, those who live in senior housing facilities report more health events and are more likely to report increases in functional limitations since wave 1. This is consistent with research that documents that relocation to such facilities is associated with the health of oneself or spouse (Choi, 1996). Residents of service-poor facilities report the highest level of chronic stressors. This is consistent with what is known about the socioeconomic and health status of those living in these facilities (see chapters 2 and 6). The findings also show that relocation to a facility since wave 1 is associated with recent stressors, specifically with chronic stressors and increases in functional limitations.

The types of stressor exposure that different residential groups report also relates in consistent ways to perceived health and personal mastery. Those who have remained in the community report the highest perceived health, high personal mastery, and significantly fewer health events and limitations (although more of other kinds of life events). However, it is important to note that sample members who live in the CCRC also report high average scores on perceived health and personal mastery, despite their more frequent experience of health events and increasing physical limitations. This does not necessarily imply that higher resource settings, such as the CCRC, may play a part in buffering the impact of health declines on the well-being of older people. It is just as likely that the characteristics and personal resources of the people who live in the CCRC—more education, higher income, a trajectory of advantage over the course of their lives—may account for this finding. What is clear is that residents of service-poor facilities face particular disadvantages that lead to greater declines in perceived health over time. Because they also experience more chronic stressors, they are also more likely to experience declines in personal mastery.

The analyses presented in this chapter have limitations that must be kept in mind. Weighting the life events measures might yield superior estimates of how stressors affect health. The measure of chronic stressors is also relatively weak. For example, it does not assess other sources of chronic stress in age-segregated housing such as more frequent exposure to deaths and illness. Relatively few study participants relocated between waves 1 and 2, making it difficult to establish whether relocation helps or hinders adjustment to stressors associated with aging. Most notably, selection into the different types of residential settings is not random in respect to exposure to health and other stressors in recent years (see also Pruchno & Rose, 2000). People may be more likely to relocate to facilities when their health declines (and if they have planned to relocate). Social status determines what type of facility an older person can afford.

Perhaps the most interesting research question for the future is whether the rates of change in perceived health and personal mastery, as well as the accumulation of stressors, will differ for those living in the service-rich and the service-poor facilities. A third wave of *Pathways* data will soon be available for analysis; it reflects another 2 years of changes in the health of *Pathways* participants. There is some indication from the first two waves of data that residents of service-poor facilities have higher rates of decline in perceived health and in mastery than do residents of the CCRC (or residents of the community). This trend has important implications for facility managers. Do the findings in this chapter suggest ways in which managers of service-poor facilities might be able to slow the rate of decline in health and mastery? Or ways in which managers of more service-rich facilities can continue to improve their programs?

It is worth noting that research on gerontology has long examined the role of personal control and mastery in maintaining the well-being of older people. For example, Krause recently noted that "Older people may live longer if they are able to maintain a sense of control over the role that is most important to them." (2000, p. 623). The findings in this chapter show that higher personal mastery is associated with increases in perceived health over time for older people. Perceived good health is associated with mortality, continued quality of life, and positive health behavior among older people (Idler & Benyamini, 1997). Streib, Falls, and LaGreca (1997), reporting on a study of 36 retirement communities, suggested that the maintenance of control and autonomy was a critical factor in increasing satisfaction and adjustment in retirement communities. How might service-poor facilities help their residents maintain a sense of mastery, control, or autonomy, even in the face of increasing health problems and losses?

Streib and his colleagues suggest four ways in which this can be done. One way is through encouragement of self-governance, including broad participation in program clubs, advisory councils, and other organizations that have input into day-to-day life in the facility. The challenge of this strategy is that as people age in place, a number will lack the energy to engage in self-governance. Another means is to help people maintain participation in meaningful activities inside or outside the facility, in activities and roles that mean the most to them (see chapter 4 of this volume). In service-poor (as well as in service-rich) facilities, the particular challenge would be to encourage continued participation by those disabled by health problems. Service-poor facilities would have the additional challenge of providing financial and other support for additional activities that would foster participation in activities, such as transportation, adequate space for meetings, and staff services. One less expensive option to encourage involvement in meaningful roles outside the facility would be to continue increasing family involvement in the facility through family councils, shared social activities, and use of facility spaces for community events involving families or service and religious groups.

Third, facility policies and programs that encourage the maintenance or improvement of individual decision-making and the sense of control over personal space may be helpful. More opportunities to personalize space (see chapter 3) would be one step. However, since many who age in place suffer from increasing functional limitations, programs to increase the feel of control or mastery over private space should probably focus on the time when new residents enter the facility.

Finally, service-poor facilities may need to think about educational programs and other types of interventions that might mitigate the impact of other chronic stressors, such as financial strains and the strains of maintaining daily activities, on the lives of their residents. For example, managers can continue to work with local service agencies and volunteer groups to provide inexpensive health maintenance programs, such as companions for walking and mild exercise, financial services, and assistance in shopping. In many larger cities (including the large city in Tompkins County), organizations such as these are already involved in such activities. In more rural areas, services and support for services may be lacking.

SUMMARY AND CONCLUSIONS

This chapter examines the distribution of and exposure to stressors in relationship to place of residence in the *Pathways* study, connecting differences in exposure to stressors with changes in perceived health and perceived mastery of life over time. Residential setting is related to exposure to stressors, with residents of facilities reporting more stressors related to health. Residents of service-poor facilities report more chronic stressors, some of which have resulted from the accumulation of social disadvantage over the course of their lives. Community residents, who are on average younger and healthier, report higher perceived health and personal mastery than do most facility residents, except for residents of the CCRC. As a group, the residents of the CCRC have maintained favorable levels of perceived health and mastery even though they have experienced increasing physical limitations and health problems. Residents of the CCRC may owe their relatively robust sense of well-being to the greater educational, financial, and social resources they have developed over the course of their lives, which enable them to cope with threats to their health more effectively than residents of the service-poor facilities.

Perhaps the most critical finding, and the one that has the most important implications for policy and practice, is that higher levels of personal mastery are associated with maintaining better perceived health over time. Thus, important targets for intervention may relate to maintaining the sense of mastery of life, as well as other activities that maintain good health behaviors.

REFERENCES

Andersson, L., & Stanich, J. (1996). Life events and their impact on health attitudes and health behavior. *Archives of Gerontology and Geriatrics, 23,* 163–177.
Aneshensel, C. S., Pearlin, L. I., Mullan, J. T., Zarit, S. H., & Whitlach, C. I. (1995). *Profiles in caregiving: The unexpected career.* New York: Academic.

Centers for Disease Control and Prevention. (2000). *Measuring healthy days*. Atlanta, GA: CDC.

Cervilla, J. A., & Prince, M. J. (1997). Cognitive impairment and social distress as different *Pathways* to depression in the elderly: A cross-sectional study. *International Journal of Geriatric Psychiatry, 12*, 995–1000.

Choi, N. G. (1996). Older persons who move: Reasons and Health Consequences. *Journal of Applied Gerontology, 15*(3), 325–344.

Chou, K., & Chi, I. (2001). Stressful life events and depressive symptoms: Social support and sense of control as mediators or moderators? *International Journal of Aging and Human Development, 52*, 155–171.

Cutrona, C., Russell, D., & Rose, J. (1986). Social support and adaptation to stress by the elderly. *Journal of Psychology and Aging, 1*, 47–54.

Evans, G. W., Wells, N. M., Chan, E., & Saltzman, H. (2001). Housing and mental health. *Journal of Consulting and Clinical Psychology, 68*, 526–530.

Glass, T. A., Kasl, S. V., & Berkman, L. (1997). Stressful life events and depressive symptoms among the elderly. *Journal of Aging and Health, 9*, 70–89.

Haug, M., Belgrave, L. L., & Gratton, B. (1984). Mental health and the elderly: Factors in stability and change over time. *Journal of Health and Social Behavior, 25*, 199–215.

Holmes, T. H., & Rahe, R. (1967). The social readjustment rating scale. *Journal of Psychosomatic Research, 11*, 213–218.

House, J. S., Umberson, D., & Landis, K. (1988). Structures and processes of social support. *Annual Review of Sociology, 14*, 293–318.

Idler, E. L., & Benyamini, Y. (1997). Self-rated health and mortality: A review of twenty-seven community studies. *Journal of Health and Social Behavior, 38*, 21–37.

Krause, N. (2000). Role-specific feelings of control and mortality. *Psychology and Aging, 15*, 617–626.

Lazarus, R. S., & Folkman, S. (1984). *Stress, appraisal, and coping*. New York: Springer.

Lefrancois, R., Leclerc, G., Hamel, S., & Gaulin, P. (2000). Stressful life events and psychological distress of the very old: Does social support have a moderating effect? *Archives of Gerontology and Geriatrics, 31*, 243–255.

Lepore, S. J. (1995). The measurement of chronic stressors. In S. Cohen, R. C. Kessler, & L. U. Gordon (Eds.), *Measuring Stress: A guide for health and social scientists* (pp.102–120). New York: Oxford University.

Lepore, S. J., Miles, H. J., & Levy, J. S. (1997). Relation of chronic and episodic stressors in psychological distress, reactivity, and health problems. *International Journal of Behavioral Medicine, 4*, 39–59.

Murrell, S. A., & Norris, F. H. (1991). Differential social support and life change as contributors to the social class-distress relationship in older adults. *Psychology and Aging, 6*, 223–231.

Ormel, J., Oldenhinkel, A. J., & Brilman, E. I. (2001). The interplay and etiological continuity of neuroticism, difficulties, and life events in the etiology of major and subsyndromal, first, and recurrent depressive episodes in later life. *American Journal of Psychiatry, 158,* 885–891.

Pearlin, L. I., & Schooler, C. (1978). The structure of coping. *Journal of Health and Social Behavior, 19,* 2–21.

Pearlin, L. I., Lieberman, M. A., Menaghan, E. G., & Mullan, J. T. (1981). The stress process. *Journal of Health and Social Behavior, 22,* 337–356.

Pruchno, R. A., & Rose, M. S. (2000). The effects of long-term care environments on health outcomes. *The Gerontologist, 40,* 422–428.

Rowe, J., & Kahn, R. L. (1998). *Successful aging.* New York: Pantheon.

Schulz, R., & Heckhausen, J. (1996). A life span model of successful aging. *American Psychologist, 51,* 702–714.

Smith, J., & Baltes, P. (1997). Profiles of psychological functioning in old age. *Journal of Personality, 12,* 458–472.

Streib, G., Falls, W. E., & LaGreca, A. J. (1985). Autonomy, power, and decision-making in thirty-six retirement communities. *The Gerontologist, 25,* 403–409.

Wethington, E., Almeida, D., Brown, G. W., Frank, E., & Kessler, R. C. (2001). The assessment of stressor exposure. In A. Vingerhoets (Ed.), *Assessment in behavioral medicine* (pp. 113–134). New York: Taylor & Francis/Brunner-Routledge.

Wheaton, B. (1999). Social stress. In C. S. Aneshensel & J. C. Phelan (Eds.), *Handbook of the sociology of mental health* (pp. 277–300). New York: Kluwer Academic/Plenum.

CHAPTER 9

Continuity and Change in Subjective Well-Being

Alice Boyce, Elaine Wethington, and Phyllis Moen

I n this chapter we examine changes in subjective well-being across time in the *Pathways to Life Quality* longitudinal sample. We examine group differences in well-being by residential setting and investigate whether group-level changes in well-being are associated with residential settings— community housing, service-rich facilities, and service-poor facilities— and recent relocation from the community to facility residence. We also examine the association of health events, health changes, other life events, chronic stressors, and increases in physical limitations with changes in individual well-being over time, and whether residential, personal, and social resources mitigate the impact of stressors on well-being.

RELOCATION AND SUBJECTIVE WELL-BEING

One life transition that has the potential to disrupt well-being is residential relocation. Although the number of older persons who move in a typical year is very small (5%), 39% of Americans do change residences after they reach age 60 (Schafer, 2000). Health problems and growing constraints caused by health problems are the most frequently cited reasons for relocation among older adults (Choi, 1996). Many moves are also undertaken because of an underlying desire to improve or maintain quality of life.

DeJong, Wilmoth, Angel, and Cornwell (1995) described a number of different motives for moving that relate to maintaining quality of life. These motives are preserving health, living near family, marrying a new spouse, seeking affordable housing, improving the living environment, seeking retirement and community amenities, living in a more desirable climate, maintaining self-reliance, and coping with a family crisis. Moving because of a decline in health or the death of a spouse is a more stressful experience than making an amenity-driven move to a better climate, house, or neighborhood. Yet moving in and of itself, no matter what the motive, can be a disruptive life experience.

What are the effects of relocation or adaptation to a new living environment on subjective well-being? Early research by Lawton and Cohen (1974) investigated the impact of residential relocation on the psychological and social well-being of older people. Their longitudinal study compared community residents to people who relocated to senior housing. Although those who relocated experienced declines in functional health, they reported significantly greater well-being, measured as psychological morale and life satisfaction, than did those who remained in the community. Housing in senior residences appeared to buffer individuals against some of the negative effects of health decline, with psychological well-being and social involvement remaining at relatively favorable levels.

Another major study incorporated the role of preexisting resources in adaptation to relocation, albeit relocation from one community to another. Smider, Essex, and Ryff (1996) investigated short-term adaptation to relocation to another community among a sample of older women. Specifically, they hypothesized that women with greater initial resources would adapt better when confronted with the difficulties of moving. Their findings suggested that emotional responses to relocation are a function of what the individual brings to the event as well as the context in which it occurs. Higher levels of perceived mastery over the environment buffered the effects of the difficulty of the move and reduced negative emotional reactions after relocation. In addition, those who were lower in resources prior to relocation benefited the most from unexpected gains associated with the move. In a related analysis, Kling, Seltzer, and Ryff (1997) also found that the successful relocators reported greater personal mastery over time and had used active and versatile styles of coping (see Mattlin, Wethington, & Kessler, 1990) to adapt to the challenges of moving.

Previous research on relocation suggests that the effects of relocation on subjective well-being may be varied, depending on social and personal factors. This in turn implies, along with the data presented in previous chapters of this volume, that the social resources found in the senior residences could also play an important part in adaptation. Aging in place does have some advantages over residential relocation in that people are able to maintain their social networks, factors that help them preserve their quality of life and a sense of personal control (Lawler, 2001). Most older adults prefer to, and do, remain in their present homes if it is at all feasible (Schafer, 1999).

There is also a considerable amount of research evidence that the subjective well-being of older people is robust, even in the face of stressors. A great deal of research in gerontology has investigated subjective well-being in older adults. Overall, measures of well-being in older adults are generally fairly similar to those reported by younger people, suggesting that aging itself does not inevitably lead to a decline in well-being. This phenomenon has been labeled the paradox of well-being (Kunzmann, Little, & Smith, 2000). That is, at a time of life when declines in well-being would seem likely because of changes in physical health, the deaths of peers and spouses, and other stressful life events associated with aging, older people are not necessarily less happy than middle-aged or younger people. In an early longitudinal study of psychiatric symptoms and mental health, Haug, Belgrave, and Gratton (1984) found that more older people remained stable or even improved than declined on these measures over a 1-year time period. Stacey and Gatz (1991) found that both negative affect and positive affect decreased over time among older people, but that the decrease in positive affect was very modest.

Numerous explanations have been proposed for the paradox of well-being. For example, Diener and Suh (1998) suggested that older people may lower their comparison standards, enabling them to interpret their life situations in a more positive light. An alternative explanation is that older persons have implemented methods of adaptation that deal more effectively with their environments. According to Carstensen's (1995) socioemotional selectivity theory, as people age they regulate their emotions in order to maximize positive affect and minimize negative affect. Diener, Colvin, Pavot, and Allman's (1991) theory of cognitive dampening proposes that individuals learn to restrict their range of affect frequency or intensity as they age and, as a consequence, experience increased well-being. It has been suggested that gains in affect management result from preexisting personality factors (such as those that promote a sense of control) as well as from adaptations to changes in social contexts and life events (Lawton, 1996).

Studies that document decreases in subjective well-being at the individual level among older people over time implicate the effects of external life factors on well-being. Analyses of the impact of life stressors in the *Pathways* sample (see chapter 9 of this volume) show that acute and chronic stressors are associated with decreases in perceived physical health and personal mastery. Although much research points to the particular contribution of health and health-related events to well-being among older people, past research has also found that other life events are important. In a meta-analysis of 25 studies estimating the impact of negative life events on depression among people age 65 and older, Kraaij, Arensman, and Spinhoven (2002) found that the loss of significant others, severe personal illness, severe illness of significant others, and financial problems were all related to higher depression scores. In addition, experiencing a larger number of life events was related to higher depression and depressive symptoms, a finding confirmed by numerous studies (Chou & Chi, 2001; Glass, Kasl, & Berkman, 1997; Ormel, Oldehinkel, & Brilman, 2001; Stallings, Dunham, Gatz, Baker, & Bengston, 1997). Thus, one would predict that older people relocating to senior housing for health reasons in the *Pathways* sample would report a lower level of well-being because they have been exposed to more life events and other stressors in the recent past (see chapter 8). This decline in well-being is apt to be moderated or absent if the move is to a service-rich facility that offers more social and supportive resources.

RESEARCH HYPOTHESES

Based on research findings relating subjective well-being to health, life events, personal and social resources, and relocation in older people, we developed the following hypotheses:

- Hypothesis 1: Subjective well-being will differ across residential groups, with those in community housing and service-rich housing reporting higher well-being than those living in service-poor housing.
- Hypothesis 2: Subjective well-being will decline slightly over time.
- Hypothesis 3: Recent movers will show increased well-being over time.
- Hypothesis 4: Older people higher in personal mastery will experience an increase in well-being after relocation.
- Hypothesis 5: Older people higher in perceived support will show increased well-being after moving to senior facilities.

METHODS

SAMPLE

The sample used in this analysis includes 508 respondents aged 60 and older who completed the first two waves of the *Pathways* study and who had complete information on all measures of interest. They range in age from 60 to 101, with an average age of 76. Two thirds (66.5%) are women. Almost half (45.3%) are married, and 36.8% are widowed. Many in the longitudinal sample are very active, with 18.5% currently working for pay and 50% currently doing volunteer work. Most rate their health as good or excellent (85.1%), but 31.6% report the onset of a new chronic health condition within the past 2 years; 76.9% report having at least one chronic health condition that requires medication. Three quarters (75.1%) experienced at least one stressful life event in the past 2 years.

To examine whether there are differences in well-being based on the type of housing in which an older person lives residence in the (community versus residence in various types of facilities) and whether residential relocation may enhance well-being, we divided our sample into four groups, based on residential setting at wave 2. We also separately examine those who have moved to senior housing facilities between waves 1 and 2. Most members of the analysis sample (n = 340, 66.9%) live in community housing and have lived there for an extended period. The mean length of residence is 27.2 years (SD = 16.4), with a range of 2 to 75 years. The residents of the continuing care retirement community (CCRC) make up 6.9% (n = 35) of the analysis sample. The CCRC opened its doors in December 1995, so residents have lived in this setting for a relatively short time (although most are not new to the geographical area and have strong ties to the community). The mean length of residence is 3.6 years (SD = 0.8), with a range of 2 to 6 years. It is important to note that the group of CCRC residents whose data are used in this chapter is smaller than in previous chapters (see also chapter 8) because the subjective well-being measures used in these analyses were not administered to the CCRC founders.

Residents of a facility providing assisted-living services make up 5.7% of the analysis sample (n = 29). They are recent movers to the facility, which opened in 1998. The remainder are residents of service-poor facilities (20.5%, n = 104). Two of the residents in service-poor facilities have moved there since wave 1.

MEASURES

Subjective Well-Being

In this chapter we analyze changes in three separate measures of subjective well-being: positive affect, negative affect, and life satisfaction. Positive affect and negative affect (Mroczek & Kolarz, 1998), are both six-item scales introduced with the stem question, "During the past 30 days, how much of the time have you felt the following?" For positive affect, the six items are: cheerful, in good spirits, extremely happy, satisfied, full of life, and calm and peaceful. For negative affect, the individual items are: so sad nothing could cheer you up, nervous, restless or fidgety, hopeless, feeling that everything was an effort, and worthless. Response options measured the frequency of these feelings from 1 (none of the time) to 5 (all of the time). Each scale is computed as a mean, with scores ranging from 1 to 5. The mean score for positive affect is 3.6 (SD = .6) and the alpha reliability is .81. The mean score for negative affect is 1.6 (SD = .5) and alpha reliability is .70. A higher score on positive affect indicates greater well-being and a higher score on negative affect denotes less well-being.

The third measure of well-being, life satisfaction, is a single-item measure. Participants were asked to rate their life at the present time on a scale of 1 to 10, with 1 being the worst possible life they can imagine and 10 being the best possible life they can imagine. Respondents report a great deal of satisfaction with their lives, with a mean rating of 8.1 (SD = 1.7) and a range from 2.5 to 10.

Social and Psychological Resources

The multivariate analyses use four measures to assess preexisting social and psychological resources that may be associated with changes in subjective well-being over time in older people. Three of these are measures of social support and the fourth is a psychological resource.

Because prior research shows that social support is multidimensional (Murrell, Norris, & Chipley, 1992) and that it matters who provides the support (Felton & Berry, 1992), three separate indicators are used. First, we use two measures from the Social Provisions scale developed by Cutrona, Russell, and Rose (1986). The first, perceived social integration, measures a sense of belonging to a group of people who share common interests and activities (see chapter 4). The second social provision, perceived reliable alliance, measures the assurance that one can count on others for assistance under any circumstances. Both of these measures are four-item scales with scores ranging from 1 (strongly disagree) to 4 (strongly agree). Levels on both measures are very high: 3.2 for social integration (alpha = .68) and 3.4 for reliable alliance (alpha = .75). The third measure of social support used is marital and partnered status at wave 2 (1 = married or partnered, 0 = not married or partnered).

The psychological resource, personal mastery, measures sense of efficacy in carrying out goals (Pearlin & Schooler, 1978). It is a seven-item scale, with scores ranging from 1 (strongly disagree) to 4 (strongly agree) (alpha = .69). Levels of personal mastery are also fairly high, with a mean of 2.96 on a 4-point scale.

Exposure to Stressors

Four measures of stress exposure are used in these analyses: the number of health events over the past 2 years, the number of other life events over the past 2 years, the number of chronic stressors, and a dummy variable coded 1 if the participant reports an increase of two functional limitations since wave 1. The content and range of the stressor measures are described in chapter 8 of this volume (Table 8.1).

ANALYTIC STRATEGY

Analysis of variance was used to test for significant group differences in well-being across residential settings at wave 2. Paired *t*-tests within residential groups were used to test the significance of change over time in measures of well-being between waves 1 and 2. Because the group-level changes may mask a considerable amount of variation among individuals in the course of well-being over time (Krause, 1999), we also examine factors that affect individual levels of psychological adaptation. To predict individual-level changes in measures of well-being, linear regression models were conducted, with the three measures of well-being used as dependent variables. Gender and age were included as well as positive resource variables, perceived health, life stressors, and residential setting.

FINDINGS

RESIDENTIAL SETTING AND WELL-BEING

Table 9.1 presents the average levels of positive affect, negative affect, and life satisfaction for participants in both waves. The means are calculated separately for the total sample (column 1); for four residential groups (column 2; CCRC, facilities offering assisted-living services, service-poor facilities, and community housing); and for respondents who have recently relocated to facilities (column 3). Caution must be observed when interpreting the significance tests because three of the groups are very small (CCRC, assisted living facilities, and recent movers to facilities).

In order to test for differences across the four settings, analysis of variance tests were conducted for each measure of subjective well-being, and for waves 1 and 2 separately. In general, community and CCRC residents

TABLE 9.1 Well-being at Wave 1 (1998) and Wave 2 (2000), by Wave 2 Residential Setting and Relocation (Means and Paired t-tests)

	Total	CCRC	Assisted -living	Service poor	Community housing facility[b]	F ratio[a]	Recently moved to facilities
Positive affect							
1998	3.66	3.74	3.37	3.55	3.73	6.14**	3.36
2000	3.62*c	3.73	3.48	3.56	3.65**c	1.91	3.45
Negative affect							
1998	1.57	1.50	1.78	1.72	1.49	7.74***	1.77
2000	1.64***c	1.60	1.72	1.83	1.57***c	7.99***	1.69
Life satisfaction							
1998	8.10	8.64	7.42	7.53	8.31	8.67***	7.53
2000	8.13	8.47	7.59	7.84	8.29	3.88***	7.48
(n)	(508)	(35)	(29)	(104)	(340)		(28)

*** $p < .001$; ** $p < .01$; * $p < .05$.
[a] Test for significance differences across residential settings.
[b] Twenty-six subjects moved to service-rich facilities; two moved to service-poor facilities.
[c] Significance levels for paired t-tests.

report the highest level of well-being for all three measures and across both waves. In 1998 (wave 1), the groups of older people who lived in service-poor facilities and people who eventually moved to the facilities offering assisted living reported significantly lower average positive affect than did CCRC residents and those who were to remain in the community. In 2000, the relative rankings across the residential groups of average positive affect remain about the same, but the differences among the groups are no longer significant (probably because mean positive affect declines among community residents; see subsequent material).

The patterns for negative affect and life satisfaction are very similar to those for positive affect. The groups living in facilities offering assisted living or in service-poor facilities at wave 2 had reported higher negative affect and lower life satisfaction at wave 1. However, negative affect and life satisfaction are still significantly associated with residential location at wave 2. This latter finding varies from the pattern associated with positive affect.

RESIDENTIAL SETTING AND CHANGES IN SUBJECTIVE WELL-BEING

The paired t-tests comparing mean levels over time are calculated separately for each of the three measures of well-being, and across residential groups. The results are summarized in Table 9.1. The main impression derived from Table 9.1 is of continuity rather than change in well-being over time, at least at the aggregate level. As noted in the introduction to this chapter, the research literature has found changes in well-being over time to be very modest among older people. For the sample as a whole, positive affect decreased over time ($p < .05$), and negative affect increased significantly ($p < .001$). Life satisfaction remained unchanged. The same pattern holds for the older people who remained in community housing. There are no significant changes in positive or negative affect in the smaller residential groups (including the service-poor facilities), nor are the differences always in the same direction. For example, for residents in assisted-living facilities in wave 2, positive affect and life satisfaction trend up and negative affect trends down. (However, none of these changes is statistically significant.)

It is important to note here that the significant changes for the sample as a whole and for the community participants are very small. A change of .04 in positive affect (see Table 9.1, panel 1, column 1) translates into modest elevation of one of six states. These statistically significant average changes are not "significant" in the clinical sense.

RECENT RELOCATION AND WELL-BEING

Only 28 members of this analysis sample relocated to facilities between waves 1 and 2 (see Table 9.1, last column). Most ($n = 26$) relocated to a facility offering assisted living. The group size is too small and statistical power too low to detect whether the slight increase in positive affect, decrease in negative affect, and decrease in life satisfaction shown in this table represent a stable trend or change.

RESIDENTIAL SETTINGS AND CHANGES OVER TIME IN SUBJECTIVE WELL-BEING

Table 9.2 presents a series of regressions of subjective well-being on residential setting, demographic factors, life stressors, and social and personal resources. (Relocation is not included as a predictor in these analyses because it overlaps almost entirely with residence in a facility offering assisted-living services.) The wave 1 score on the measure of subjective well-being is included among the predictors. The inclusion of the wave 1 measure of well-being transforms the regression into an analysis of change in the dependent variable over time.

Column 1 presents the regression for positive affect as a dependent variable. Among the variables indicating residential setting, only living in the CCRC is associated with a marginal increase ($b = .160$, $p < .10$). The excluded residential category is living in the community. This coefficient suggests that CCRC dwellers are slightly more likely to show an increase in positive affect than are people who remain in the community. Having more education is associated with decreases in positive affect over time ($b = -.044$, $p < .05$). Recent health events are not significantly related to

TABLE 9.2 Regression of Well-being at Wave 2 on Residential Setting, Life Stressors, and Social and Personal Resources

	Positive affect	Negative affect	Life satisfaction
	b	b	b
Well-being, W1	.483***	.422***	.288***
Age	.003	.030	.022*
Female	−.007	.009	.094
Education	−.094**	.039	.093
Married	.060	.038	.437**
Lives in CCRC, W2[a]	.160+	.015	.069
Lives in assisted living, W2[a]	.019	.029	−.663
Lives in service-poor facility, W2[a]	.042	.164**	.158
Health events	−.031	.004	−.176*
Other life events	−.029+	.021	−.094+
Chronic stressors	−.097	.009	−.312*
Increase in functional limitations, W1–W2	−.181*	.138**	−.008
Perceived physical health, W1	.022	−.047+	.007
Social integration, W1	.070	.009	.373+
Reliable alliance, W1	.133*	−.056	.160
Personal mastery, W1	.043	−.086	.364+
Intercept	1.02**	1.57***	1.54
F ratio	18.02***	14.76***	9.00**
R^2	.39	.34	.24
R^2 (adjusted)	.36	.32	.21

*** $p < .001$; ** $p < .01$; * $p < .05$
[a] The excluded residential setting is community housing.
W1, wave 1; W2, wave 2.

changes in positive affect, although an increase in limitations is associated with a decrease in positive affect ($b = -.181, p < .05$). Other life events are marginally associated with decreases in positive affect ($b = -.029, p < 10$). Reliable alliance is the only social or personal resource significantly related to increases in positive affect over time ($b = .133, p < .05$).

Column 2 displays the same sets of predictors, with changes in negative affect as the outcome. Those who live in service-poor facilities are more likely than community residents to show increases in negative affect ($b = .164, p < .01$). Increases in negative affect are also significantly associated with an increase in limitations since wave 1 ($b = .138, p < .01$) and with having poorer perceived health at wave 1 ($b = -.047, p < .10$).

The regression for life satisfaction is presented in column 3. No residential setting seems to be associated with different rates of changes over time. Age ($b = .022, p < .05$) and being married ($b = .437, p < .01$) are associated with increases in life satisfaction across time. Health events ($b = -.176, p < .05$), other life events ($b = -.094, p < .10$), and chronic stressors ($b = -.312, p < .05$) are associated with decreases in life satisfaction. Social integration ($b = .373, p < .10$) and personal mastery ($b = .364, p < .10$) are associated with marginal increases in life satisfaction over time.

RELOCATION, PERSONAL MASTERY, AND WELL-BEING

In general, a higher score on personal mastery at wave 1 does not predict an increase in well-being at wave 2 (see Table 9.2). Higher personal mastery is associated with a marginal ($p < .10$) increase in life satisfaction at wave 2, but it is not at all associated with changes in negative or positive affect across time. (This is in contrast to findings in chapter 8, where higher personal mastery at wave 1 is associated with increases in perceived health at wave 2). We hypothesized specifically that people higher in personal mastery would adjust better after relocation. In order to test this hypothesis we conducted a test for the interaction of personal mastery with recently moving to a facility. However, this interaction is not significant. Since most residents of the CCRC and the facilities offering assisted living are not long-term residents, we also estimated interaction terms between living in these settings and personal mastery at wave 1. None of these interaction terms are significant. We therefore reject the hypothesis that personal mastery is associated with greater well-being after relocation to a facility.

RELOCATION, SOCIAL SUPPORT, AND WELL-BEING

Higher levels of social support at wave 1 are not consistently related to increases in subjective well-being over time. Reliable alliance is significantly related to increases in positive affect ($b = .133$, $p < .05$). Social integration is marginally related to increases in life satisfaction ($b = .373$, $p < .10$). Neither is significantly related to decreases in negative affect. Marital status is related to increases in life satisfaction at wave 2 ($b = .437$, $p < .01$). We hypothesized specifically that people higher in social support would adjust better after relocation. We tested a series of interactions between recent relocation and the three measures of social support. However, none of the tested interactions are significant. Preexisting levels of social support are not associated with greater increases in well-being after relocation to a facility.

IMPLICATIONS FOR RESEARCH, POLICY, AND PRACTICE

In this chapter we examine group and individual changes in subjective well-being across time in the *Pathways to Life Quality* longitudinal sample. We examine group differences in well-being by residential setting and investigate whether changes in well-being are associated with residential settings—community housing, service-rich facilities, and service-poor facilities—and recent relocation from the community to facility residence. We also examine the association of health events, other life events, chronic stressors, and increases in physical limitations with changes in individual well-being over time, and whether residential, personal, and social resources mitigate the impact of stressors on well-being.

There are significant group differences in subjective well-being by residential setting at wave 2. Those changes, however, are almost all the consequence of stability in preexisting differences in well-being between the residential groups, measured at wave 1. We do not find strong evidence that senior housing facilities enhance well-being (see also Pruchno & Rose, 2000), although it is likely that residences with more services play a role in maintaining the high level of well-being of people who move there. Rather, we find that different types of people live in different types of settings. In particular, we find that people whose declining health attracts them to facilities that offer assisted-living services have lower well-being at wave 1. We also find that residents of service-poor facilities report lower average well-being at both time points. On the whole, subjective well-being remains remarkably stable across time at the group level.

We also examine the impact of recent relocation on individual well-being, and the role of personal and social resources in promoting better adaptation to the difficulties of relocation. We find no evidence that higher levels of personal mastery before the move promote better adaptation to relocation, at least for the measures of well-being used in these analyses. Nor does higher mastery at wave 1 predict increased well-being at wave 2, independent of residential setting.

It is worth noting that previous research into the role of personal mastery and relocation did not look specifically at the type of population represented in the *Pathways* study. The relocaters in the *Pathways* study are older (the average age of those who relocated between waves 1 and 2 is 81 years) and have been suffering from increasing mobility limitations (see chapter 6).

Preexisting social resources also are not consistently related to better adaptation after relocation. Social integration and reliable alliance are marginally related to increases in well-being in the sample as whole. The married or partnered, however, do report significantly higher life satisfaction in the sample as a whole. Yet none of these three social resources buffer the impact of relocation on well-being.

Perhaps the most important finding in this chapter is how resilient and robust older people are in periods of life transition. As noted earlier, relocation does not appear to be related to declines in well-being. Nor do life events and stressors produce long-lasting changes in well-being. Exposure to stressors is associated with changes in life satisfaction over time, but it is not strongly associated with longitudinal changes in positive and negative affect. The overall findings suggest a success story: For many aspects of subjective well-being, older people are very resilient through change.

Do these findings on the continuity of well-being over time have implications for facility managers and planners? There are three important implications. First, movers to facilities may often have much lower levels of subjective well-being than other people their age, as well as poorer physical health and mobility. Second, service-rich facilities attract people with higher levels of well-being than do service-poor facilities. Third, movers to service-rich facilities have better resources for coping with increasing health problems and probably make more efficient use of services.

Programs to assist adjustment to senior housing facilities may benefit greatly from acknowledging that well-being is declining along with health at this time. Certainly the expectation (and justification) for housing developments that offer assisted-living services is that these services will contribute to enhanced quality of life by reducing the strains of daily living. Yet this study and another study comparing older people who relocated to either a skilled nursing facility or to assisted living (Pruchno & Rose, 2000) have not found strong evidence that assisted-living services significantly increase psychological well-being. Given the known relationship between preexisting psychological well-being and changes in health over time (see chapter 8 of this volume), programs to aid readjustment should target the maintenance of well-being as well as assistance for health.

The significant preexisting differences we have found among residential groups also suggests that different types of facilities will need to adopt different types of programs. No one set of interventions will work for every facility because the populations will be different. For example, the residents of the CCRC have much higher levels of education, income, and occupational attainment than do the residents of the service-poor facilities. An educational or informational program designed to assist the residents of the CCRC would not transfer to more conventional types of congregate housing, if only because informational messages must be keyed to the needs of a group in order to be persuasive. Similarly, support interventions developed in a service-poor setting to increase levels of satisfaction and positive affect would not necessarily translate to a more service-rich facility. Norms that guide the appropriateness of accepting help and support differ across educational groups and may affect the effectiveness of a support intervention (Cohen, Gottlieb, & Underwood, 2000).

The findings in this chapter also suggest that in service-rich settings such as a CCRC, the preexisting coping skills of the residents are higher. This is undoubtedly because the residents of this facility have benefited from social and economic advantages all of their lives. No set of programs at a facility can help older people overcome a lifetime of disadvantage. However, educational and informational programs about the issues surrounding aging can help people cope with managing chronic disease and relationship losses.

The challenge for facility managers and planners, however, is how to provide useful and appropriate services in low-resource facilities in which neither the facility nor the residents can pay for these services. One way to begin addressing this challenge is to connect residents in senior housing with services available in the community. Isolation of senior housing from community life compounds the difficulties for residents, whose well-being is compromised. Particularly in smaller towns and in rural areas, senior housing centers could be located near churches (offering social facilities and the ability to maintain informal social contacts), schools (offering recreational facilities and the benefits of intergenerational interaction), and transportation and shopping hubs (offering access to community services).

SUMMARY AND CONCLUSIONS

The major conclusion of this chapter is that the subjective well-being of older people is robust and resilient through life transitions, including relocation to a senior facility. Yet the well-being of older people varies according to their educational, financial, and life histories. Although no facility can overcome an individual's life time of disadvantage, managers and planners of senior housing facilities should recognize the diversity of experiences that older people bring to these facilities. They should also recognize that facilities that offer fewer services and are affordable to low-income seniors disproportionately attract residents with diminished subjective well-being. An individual's level of subjective well-being may have an impact on how effectively he or she utilizes services available in the community and in the facility.

REFERENCES

Carstensen, L. L. (1995). Evidence for a life-span theory of socioemotional selectivity. *Current Directions in Psychological Science, 4*, 151–155.

Choi, N. G. (1996). Older persons who move: Reasons and health consequences. *Journal of Applied Gerontology, 15*, 325–344.

Chou, K., & Chi, I. (2001). Stressful life events and depressive symptoms: Social support and sense of control as mediators or moderators. *International Journal of Aging and Human Development, 52*, 155–171.

Cohen, S., Gottlieb, B. H., & Underwood, L. G. (2000). Social relationships and health. In S. Cohen, L. G. Underwood, & B. H. Gottlieb (Eds.), *Social support measurement and intervention: A guide for health and social scientists* (pp. 3–28). New York: Oxford University.

Cutrona, C., Russell, D., & Rose, J. (1986). Social support and adaptation to stress by the elderly. *Journal of Psychology and Aging, 1*, 47–54.

DeJong, G. F., Wilmoth, J. M., Angel, J. L., & Cornwell, G. T. (1995). Motives and the geographic mobility of very old Americans. *Journal of Gerontology, 50B*, S395–S404.

Diener, E., Colvin, C. R., Pavot, W. G., & Allman, A. (1991). The psychic costs of intense positive affect. *Journal of Personality and Social Psychology, 61*, 492–503.

Diener, E,. & Suh, M. E. (1998). Subjective well-being and age: An international analysis. In K. W. Schaie and M. P. Lawton (Eds.), *Annual review of gerontology and geriatrics, focus on emotion and adult development* (Vol. 17, pp. 304–325). New York: Springer.

Felton, B. J., & Berry C. A. (1992). Do the sources of the urban elderly's social support determine its psychological consequences? *Psychology and Aging, 7*, 89–97.

Glass, T. A., Kasl, S. V., & Berkman, L. (1997). Stressful life events and depressive symptoms among the elderly. *Journal of Aging and Health, 9*, 70–89.

Haug, M., Belgrave, L. L., & Gratton, B. (1984). Mental health and the elderly: Factors in stability and change over time. *Journal of Health and Social Behavior, 25*, 100–115.

Heidrich, S. M., & Ryff, C. D. (1993). Physical and mental health in later life: The self-system as mediator. *Psychology and Aging, 8*, 327–338.

Kling, K. C., Seltzer, M. M., & Ryff, C. D. (1997). Distinctive late-life challenges: Implications for coping and well-being. *Psychology and Aging, 12*, 288–295.

Kraaij, V., Arensman, E., & Spinhoven, P. (2002). Negative life events and depression in elderly persons: A meta-analysis. *Journal of Gerontology, 57B*, P87–P94.

Krause, N. (1999). Assessing change in social support during late life. *Research on Aging, 21*, 539–569.

Kunzmann, U., Little, T. D., & Smith, J. (2000). Is age-related stability of subjective well-being a paradox? Cross-sectional and longitudinal evidence from the Berlin Aging Study. *Psychology and Aging, 15*, 511–526.

Lawler, K. (2001). *Aging in place: Coordinating housing and health care provision for America's growing elderly population.* Cambridge, MA: Joint Center for Housing Studies of Harvard University.

Lawton, M. P. (1996). Quality of life and affect in later life. In C. Magai & S. H. McFadden (Eds.), *Handbook of emotion, adult development and aging* (pp. 327–348). San Diego, CA: Academic.

Lawton, M. P., & Cohen, J. (1974). The generality of housing impact on the well-being of older people. *Journal of Gerontology, 29*, 194–204.

Mattlin, J., Wethington, E., & Kessler, R. C. 1990. Situational determinants of coping and coping effectiveness. *Journal of Health and Social Behavior, 31*, 103–122.

Mroczek, D. K., & Kolarz, C. M. (1998). The effect of age on positive and negative affect: A developmental perspective on happiness. *Journal of Personality and Social Psychology, 75*, 1333–1349.

Murrell, S. A., Norris, F. H., & Chipley, Q. T. (1992). Functional versus structural support, desirable events, and positive affect in older adults. *Psychology and Aging, 7*, 562–570.

Ormel, J., Oldehinkel, A. J., & Brilman, E. I. (2001). The interplay and etiological continuity of neuroticism, difficulties, and life events in the etiology of major and subsyndromal, first, and recurrent depressive episodes in later life. *American Journal of Psychiatry, 158*, 885–891.

Pearlin, L. I., & Schooler, C (1978). The structure of coping. *Journal of Health and Social Behavior, 19*, 2–21.

Pruchno, R. A., & Rose, M. S. (2000). The effect of long-term care environments on health outcomes. *The Gerontologist, 40*, 422–428.

Schafer, R. (2000). *Housing America's seniors.* Cambridge, MA: Joint Center for Housing Studies of Harvard University.

Schafer, R. (1999). *Housing America's elderly population.* Cambridge, MA: Joint Center for Housing Studies of Harvard University, Working Paper Series.

Smider, N. A., Essex, M. J., & Ryff, C. D. (1996). Adaptation to community relocation: The interactive influence of psychological resources and contextual factors. *Psychology and Aging, 11*, 362–372.

Stacey, C. A., & Gatz, M. (1991). Cross-sectional age differences and longitudinal change on the Bradburn Affect Balance Scale. *Journals of Gerontology, 46*, P76–P78.

Stallings, M. C., Dunham, C. C., Gatz, M., Baker, L. A., & Bengtson, V. L. (1997). Relationships among life events and psychological well-being: More evidence for a two-factor theory of well-being. *Journal of Applied Gerontology, 16*, 104–119.

SECTION 6

Conclusion

CHAPTER 10

Lessons for Providers and Consumers

John A. Krout and Karl Pillemer

The notion of *home* is an extraordinarily powerful one for many older persons. Adult children often commiserate with one another about their parents' reluctance to leave a living situation that has become isolating, hazardous, or too difficult to maintain. What appears to be a straightforward and rational decision—the move to a supportive living arrangement—can be met by fierce resistance from an older parent determined to remain independent and in a familiar setting.

One of the most evocative representations of the need for a real home at the end of life is the film *The Trip to Bountiful*. In the film, the elderly Mrs. Watts (in an Oscar-winning performance by Geraldine Paige) lives in a tiny apartment with her son and daughter-in-law. Forced to sleep on the living room couch, nagged and badgered by her daughter-in-law, Mrs. Watts is despondent and depressed. She longs to return to her beloved childhood home, imagining she can live independently in this idealized situation. After escaping and making the trip back home, the dilapidated, deserted house provides a stark return to reality, and the end to her fantasies about independent living.

Both that remarkable movie and this book point to similar truths about aging and the importance of living environments. It has now become commonplace to highlight the positive aspects of "successful aging." Indeed, this volume points out a number of factors that lead to well-being, social integration, and life satisfaction in the later years. However, it is also unfortunately true that many people spend the final stages of their lives with a serious burden of chronic illness or disability. In such situations, older persons and their families face a number of stressful and difficult decisions,

197

many of which revolve around the question "Where will I live when I can no longer meet all of my own needs?"

This question and the issues it raises reflect one of the grand themes in social gerontology during the past 50 years: the conflict between dependency and autonomy in later life (Cohler, 1983; Luescher & Pillemer, 1998). Negotiating the ambivalence between increasing needs for help and support from others on the one hand and the desire to remain independent and in control of one's life on the other is one of the key dynamics of the aging process. It is in its potential to alleviate the dilemma between dependence and autonomy that supportive living arrangements play such a critical role. By changing the living environment and providing a new context for daily activities, housing has the potential to promote autonomy, foster physical and psychological well-being, and relieve pressure on caregiving family members.

As the chapters in this volume clearly demonstrate, however, that potential has not yet been realized. Housing for older persons appears to be a "many-splintered thing," in which resources are not necessarily matched to the needs of older persons; in which amenities tend to be distributed according to socioeconomic status; and in which older persons' planning for residential moves is often limited. This is problematic because the authors also show the tremendous potential of appropriate and enriched housing to improve the quality of later life.

The *Pathways to Life Quality* study addresses these issues in a multi-faceted way. Using an in-depth study of a small region, investigators were able to examine the relationship between where older people live and their quality of life. Further, the study was able to provide unique information on the way in which older persons make residential decisions. The rich data that the study produced led to a number of important implications for practice and policy, which we detail in this chapter.

CONSIDERATIONS IN DEVELOPING POLICY AND PRACTICE RECOMMENDATIONS

Prior to discussing specific implications, it is worthwhile to make several observations based on the findings reported in this book. These observations provide the context for recommendations for housing policy and practice as well for older adults and their families as they plan for housing needs in later life. In particular, we note that the research reported in this volume has revealed four major points regarding residential options and decision making that are relevant to the question "What should our society do in regard to housing for older persons?"

RESIDENTIAL DECISIONS MUST BE CONSIDERED USING A DYNAMIC, LIFE COURSE PERSPECTIVE

The contributions to this volume clearly demonstrate the value of the life course perspective. This perspective highlights the dynamic nature of roles and living circumstances as individuals age. The life course perspective focuses our attention on situational imperatives confronting families, on the possibilities for personal change during critical transitions, and on the adjustments individuals must make to changing circumstances. Thus, individual lives can be seen as consisting of shifts in relationships, roles, and identities over time, with concomitant shifts in vulnerabilities and resources and, consequently, in housing needs. As Moen and colleagues note in chapter 9, later life is a time of both gains and losses in a variety of domains.

Following the life course perspective, Erickson and Moen note in chapter 5 that residential location should be seen not as a static ecological address, but rather as a process of transition for older persons. As their research shows, the transition into a congregate facility can have both positive and negative consequences for individuals, with an increased sense of personal security but also a reduced sense of psychological integration into the community. This volume shows the limitations of viewing housing as a "snapshot," in which individuals are understood only in their current setting. Instead, the *Pathways* study portrays housing in later life as a dynamic, fluid situation, in which individuals consider alternatives; plan—sometimes for years—to move into a new setting; consider home modifications; and actually move into and out of various types of living arrangements. Both policymakers and practitioners must take this dynamic situation into consideration.

CONTEXT MATTERS

The second observation relates to the key importance of contextual factors in determining individual adjustment, well-being, and life satisfaction. The contexts and environments in which people grow old dramatically affect their experiences. As this book makes abundantly clear, the physical and social characteristics of the housing environment are related to various outcomes for older persons and some clearly are related to more positive levels of well-being than others. In our study, older adults living in residential environments with more amenities generally report higher levels of psychological well-being. Residents of senior housing, in general, report more health problems than those living in noncongregate settings, partly because their health problems make it difficult for them to live more independently. We attribute a significant number of these differences to compositional effects (sociodemographic differences individuals bring with them) and life course experiences such as past health behaviors and illnesses and previous access to services. Given the short, 2-year time frame of the analyses reported here, it is very difficult to determine the impact of a given residential environment, net other factors, on well-being. As data are collected in future cycles, we will be better able to measure changes from the baseline that will help us examine this question.

But regardless of the cause, well-being profiles and service needs do differ based on an older adult's living environment and this has implications for the social dynamics of those environments, including interactions among residents and between residents and staff. This fact also has implications for housing and service policy issues and for families faced with making decisions about housing options for older relatives. We also observe that, compared to longer term congregate housing residents, those who have moved in recently initially experience a period of adjustment in social relationships and psychological well-being that also has implications for practice and policy.

Recognizing that particular ecologies are more supportive to older persons is, in fact, a positive and hopeful sign. It focuses greater attention on a factor that generally has been ignored in studies of the health and psychological well-being of older adults. This focus is particularly needed as options such as assisted living and CCRCs expand to meet the housing needs and preferences of older adults. Clearly, enriching and expanding housing contexts is a promising way to enhance the lives of older adults.

HOUSING REFLECTS CUMULATIVE ADVANTAGE OR DISADVANTAGE

Decades of research have made it clear that people who are advantaged in one area of life tend also to have advantages in other domains of life. For example, persons with higher incomes tend to be in better health, to have had more rewarding careers, and to have more extensive social roles and relationships. A lifetime of advantage or disadvantage is clearly reflected in the research on housing presented in this volume. Although new options for assisted living and life care are burgeoning, such options are generally available only to persons who have much higher-than-average incomes. Some states do provide assisted living for lower income persons through the use of Medicaid waivers and other public monies, but the number of older adults who have their housing needs met in this way is small. The fact is that good assisted living and life care are expensive, and lower income adults generally have little access to them. In-home care is another option, but the money available to the economically disadvantaged for this type of service is minuscule compared to that which is directed to traditional nursing home care. Many housing options for lower income individuals are generally relegated to the nonprofit sector and are dependent on community generosity, tenuous governmental support, and systems of family and informal care. Solutions must be found for this situation, or housing arrangements for older persons will continue the accumulation of disadvantage among persons who are the most vulnerable.

THE HETEROGENEITY OF THE OLDER POPULATION MUST BE RECOGNIZED

Perhaps the clearest message to emerge from the *Pathways* study is the danger of generalizing about "the elderly" with regard to housing decisions. In fact, each chapter in this book has revealed considerable heterogeneity in this sample of older persons. They differ considerably in their attitudes toward housing options, their individual preferences, the degree to which they plan ahead for increasing dependency needs, and their views about what makes for good housing design. Any policy and practice recommendations must acknowledge the wide range of individual differences among older persons as they make housing transitions. One-size-fits-all solutions will simply not work, given the vast individual differences in backgrounds, personality characteristics, life experiences, and preferences of the older population.

IMPLICATIONS FOR POLICY AND PRACTICE

With these overarching observations as a background, what are some priorities for policy and practice that emerge from the *Pathways* data? The findings detailed in this volume point to several pressing needs.

ATTENTION MUST BE DIRECTED TO THOSE WITH AN ACCUMULATION OF DISADVANTAGE

It is not surprising that our analyses revealed that those having higher levels of disability reside in subsidized housing environments as opposed to other settings. We found that senior apartment (service-poor) residents suffer more from serious health conditions such as heart conditions and diabetes, have the lowest levels of education and income, are typically not married, and have poorer health behaviors. Obviously, individual demographic and behavioral characteristics account for this disadvantage and may be very difficult to change. Unfortunately, lower income housing often has few (if any) on-site services that enable residents to live independently for a longer time. To avoid excess disability and a diminishing quality of life for persons with an accumulation of disadvantage, several steps are indicated by the *Pathways* research.

One response is to find ways to increase the availability of services on-site, targeted to the most prevalent health problems of the population living there. Perhaps on-site staff could be trained to provide some of these services. Another, and probably more feasible, approach may be to develop arrangements with local hospitals, county departments of health or offices for aging to conduct screenings, education, or intervention programs. Informal buddy-system networks with professional training and support might serve as another complementary approach.

Given their poorer health, many lower income senior housing residents could benefit from working with social workers or other professionals who could assist them through referrals to services or act as care managers. Older adults living in rural housing, for example, generally have less access to services, and budgets for these facilities are often small with only part-time on-site managers with little background in services. One strategy for meeting the needs of such residents would be to have circuit-riding care coordinators make scheduled visits to meet with residents and make referrals to services in the community. Information and referral programs could also make targeted efforts to reach senior housing residents. Considering that working with congregate populations brings some economies of scale, these approaches would seem to make sense from both policy and budgetary perspectives.

COMMUNITY-BASED SERVICES SHOULD BE BETTER INTEGRATED WITH HOUSING

Our data show that community-based service utilization varies considerably depending on the service. Respondents are most likely to report using senior centers and transportation services, followed by home health and homemaker services. However, we found that usage rates also vary widely depending on where a person lives. Community residents were least likely to use services, perhaps because they were younger and because a selection effect results in those less able to live independently moving to congregate housing. Our data do show that residents of service-poor housing are generally more likely to use services because their need is greater. This appears to be an appropriate match of service use and need. However, often community-based service providers do not adequately target senior housing residents for services because it is assumed their needs are met as part of their housing. In fact, unless congregate housing is specifically designed for and reimbursed for providing supportive services, these services are not made available to residents.

This underlies the broader issue of the lack of integration of housing and services for older adults in the United States. Historically, housing and services have been planned, implemented, funded, and regulated by different organizations and agencies. Housing has been largely a private-sector, for-profit product, whereas community-based services have been much more likely to reside in the government and not-for-profit arenas. The needs of seniors, as illustrated in the research reported here, cannot be very well served by such a situation. A better approach lies in planning and designing congregate housing with the expectation that the need for health and social supportive services will emerge for many residents over time, rather than ignoring this eventuality or assuming that these needs will somehow be met by informal supports.

Remember that we found that respondents who had recently moved to congregate housing generally reported higher rates of service use. We would expect this because moving to such housing is often associated with push factors such as declining health and the need for more support. However, we found a mixed bag when it came to service use pre- and post-move. Homemaker service and referral use went up, suggesting that some community-based services continued to be accessed. But senior center attendance declined considerably even as transportation use remained, in aggregate, about the same. This finding might be a cause for concern as the senior center in the county offers a wide range of education and wellness programs as well as opportunities for social engagement. Why did the movers not stay connected with the senior center? Perhaps staff there was unaware of the move or perhaps the movers had experienced a loss of interest in center programs. Whatever the reason, this situation would appear to be one that could be remedied without major investment of resources. A phone call from an outreach worker or "friendly visitor" could serve to keep or reestablish a connection between the mover and the programs in which he or she had participated.

Our findings on change in the use of service both in the aggregate and by individuals also help to establish what many service providers know— service use and users are fluid and variable. This is a reality that takes time, money, and expertise to respond to and needs to be recognized in budgets and funding streams. Home health and homemaker services show the largest changes in overall use over time and this volatility can make planning for staffing and other resources more difficult. These services, in particular, might benefit from flexible and responsive program operation and priorities, staffing, and budgeting. Utilization of other services such as senior centers, home delivered meals, and legal assistance remained unchanged overall, so one could argue that these services would face less difficulty in planning for resources over time

Other implications of the data are found in the variation in service utilization in the variety of housing arrangements of the older adults in our sample. Assuming that the use levels reflect service need, it is clear that such need varies considerably according to the type of housing arrangement. Based on our findings, managers of congregate housing (especially those with few on-site services and small professional staffs) should plan to provide information or links to specific services (or provide them on-site) that are most appropriate for growing needs as residents age in place. Our findings also suggest that programs could be developed to decrease the conditions that lead to the need for service use.

ATTENTION TO ADJUSTMENT NEEDS OF MOVERS IS NECESSARY

When we compared recent movers to congregate living to longer term residents, we found that newer residents appear to experience an initial period of social adjustment and feelings of lessened social involvement and integration. Indeed, this pattern appears to be normative and is important because these aspects of social support can be related to both life satisfaction and health. To avoid or lessen these experiences, facility staff could systematically prepare incoming residents for this experience, and thus allow them to anticipate it. Staff could also plan activities to reduce the length and impact of the adjustment process. A number of strategies could be attempted: more information about this likely change and how to counter it given to new arrivals and their family members; formal welcoming activities; a buddy system that links new residents with longer term ones; communication with family members, where available, to help staff identify new residents who might be having difficulty in their adjustment; and, where common dining facilities are used, making sure staff are aware of and responsive to new arrivals.

Our findings demonstrate that there is considerable variation in the levels of satisfaction, social participation and integration, health, and other measures of well-being of residents of the various senior housing facilities. We cannot determine the relative degree to which these differences reflect variation in the characteristics of older adults living in different settings as opposed to how living in those settings impacts the residents. But we can say that these differences suggest that the resource, staff training, and program needs of various senior housing facilities cannot be addressed through "one size fits all" responses.

ACCURATE AND CURRENT INFORMATION IS NEEDED REGARDING LIVING ARRANGEMENTS

National surveys have shown that older people and their families generally have very little understanding of congregate residential options, the services that are provided in them, and the quality-of-life issues that might be affected by moving. Older adults tend to seek out information when the need to move arises, and that need can develop suddenly. People who move to CCRCs tend to be exceptions to that rule because this housing option requires a very large financial investment and generally involves the selling of a primary residence that has been lived in for many years. Our research supports these generalizations and the need for a greater emphasis on educating older adults about the kinds of housing options available, what can be expected during and after a move, and the challenges and changes that can arise when one ages in place in a variety of settings.

Pathways findings on moving expectations and anticipated living arrangements are instructive on this issue. For example, aging in place is by far the most commonly anticipated future living arrangement in our sample, yet older people, and many professionals, generally have very little understanding of issues such as home modification. People living in senior housing can face restrictions on how long they can stay there once their health declines, and the assumption that they can live there as long as they want is often incorrect. Public monies for home modifications are very limited and modifications can be very expensive. Relocation to senior housing, on the other hand, can involve large financial decisions and significant psychological issues as people leave behind houses and neighborhoods that have tremendous meaning and importance to their lives and those of their children and even their grandchildren. Our findings clearly suggest that changes in social relationships and psychological well-being can occur as people move away from, or sometimes toward, friends and family. Congregate facilities have social dynamics that can be very different from the ones older people are accustomed to.

Educating older adults and their families about these issues should be more than a matter of personal responsibility. Aging service providers and housing professionals (including practitioners, builders, developers, and funders) in the public, non-for-profit, and private sectors should work together to provide information on relocation and housing issues. National advocacy groups such as AARP and the National Council on the Aging could also play an important role, as could public service announcements on radio and television. What kind of information should be disseminated? Topics could include the availability and cost of housing options; agencies that can provide information on these options; professionals who can provide advice on moving and home modifications; the kinds of social and psychological changes that can accompany a move; and common home modifications that can facilitate aging in place. One approach would be to develop a housing kit (and a web site) with materials written in easily understood language and a checklist of questions that should be asked and answered before the decision to move is made.

Providing this type of information will require a considerable investment in developing materials and educating professionals to use them effectively. In addition to a knowledge gap among consumers, a knowledge gap also exists among many who work in aging and in housing policy and practice. One must also recognize the lack of availability of affordable housing options in many areas and consider the appropriateness of providing information about options that are not available locally or are accessible only to those with considerable financial and social resources.

STEPS MUST BE TAKEN TO PREVENT THE PROGRESSION OF DISABILITY AMONG CONGREGATE HOUSING RESIDENTS

Our findings, in general, indicate that residents of congregate facilities appear not to age in place as well as those living in the community. Certainly there is a strong selection effect operating here and we would expect that people often move to congregate facilities precisely because of declining health or other situations that make it more difficult for them to live more independently.

Chronic conditions reflect the cumulative impact of many factors such as health behaviors over many years. They do not result from living for a few years in one setting as opposed to another. Residents living in senior housing have spent many more years living in a variety of non-senior housing environments. Thus, our findings obviously do not demonstrate that housing causes the observed chronic conditions. Nonetheless, from the perspective of practice and policy, these findings are important because they document differences in health and disability of the residents of various housing arrangements and underscore the fact that chronic illness is found in residents of all types of housing. Thus, treatment, education, and prevention activities are needed in all of them.

Whatever the reason, the facts that congregate housing residents are less healthy and have greater functional impairment have implications for housing staff. Ideally, facilities' staffs can provide wellness programs and encourage wellness-promoting behaviors. If resources are not available to support formal programming, staff can provide information on wellness and wellness programs that are available in the community. Once residents' health and social needs have been identified, staff members should have information they can distribute concerning available community services. This function could also be performed by select residents who are trained by community agencies to act as volunteers or are paid as peer counselors. Residents and staff need to have information about community services and how residents can access them. Where possible, housing practitioners should be able to respond to each individual resident's needs, as these needs can be very different from one person to the next. Likewise, since facilities are different from each other, their resource, staff training, and program needs are different. Plans and programs to respond to resident needs are best if they are tailored to specific types of facilities and their populations.

TOWARD A VISION OF THE FUTURE

When making concrete policy and practice recommendations, it is necessary to consider the constraints placed on the range of options, caused typically by a lack of public and private funding for possible programs. However, it is also instructive to speculate at the conclusion of this chapter on the characteristics of a system of housing options for older persons in America that better meets the needs of all older adults. That is, what would the optimal configuration and operation of housing arrangements be in a given geographic area? Several features of this system are clearly indicated by the *Pathways* findings.

A WIDE RANGE OF OPTIONS IS NEEDED

Ideally, a continuum of housing options would exist in the community to meet the family situations, functional status, and personal preferences of all older persons. These options range from the least restrictive setting (that which provides the greatest autonomy) to the most restrictive (that required by persons with the greatest dependency needs). Options in such a continuum would include: living in one's own home (with or without physical modifications); living at home receiving care from family members or professionals; senior housing; assisted living; and nursing homes. Some environments may have more than one of these alternatives or, like CCRCs, have all of them.

This continuum is misleading in the sense that it suggests a progression of housing options that older adults might move through when, in fact, most older adults are likely to experience only one, or all of the first three. Additionally, many older adults suffer acute health problems that move them from living at home directly to assisted living or a nursing home. Sometimes this occurs because of the lack of availability or affordability of the middle options. Thus, perhaps the word *menu* is more appropriate than *continuum*.

Availability and affordability (another dimension of accessibility) are the key aspects of a preferred system and they are the major challenges, given the existing system of long-term care policy, funding, and regulation in America. Medicare and Medicaid help ensure widespread access to traditional nursing home care for those who are 65 or older and have low incomes. But access to the other options is not ensured. And nursing home care in America is based on a hospital model not on a community-based model in which persons needing care can receive it while living in traditional home-like environments. Resource issues probably mean that not every community can have the full range of housing options, but every older American should have reasonable access to affordable housing options.

A model that would better fit with the preferences and expectations of older adults in America would have a much heavier emphasis on home care by professionals, affordable congregate options for those not needing considerable skilled care, and the delivery of skilled care in settings that are more closely integrated into neighborhoods and not institutional in design or operation. Such approaches are fairly common in Western Europe (Regnier, 1994).

In addition, the options for older adults that currently dominate the American housing landscape are fragmented and not coordinated. Furthermore, housing has traditionally not been well integrated with other services. In fact, housing is generally not seen as a service, but rather as a brick-and-mortar issue. Often, older adults who are moved to nursing homes stop receiving the community-based services they had been getting, not because the need has diminished, but because of a bias against serving nursing home residents and because the policies of community-based service programs often require it. A better approach would institute greater coordination and communication between housing and other service providers.

INFORMATION AND REFERRAL ARE NEEDED

Services that link older persons with the range of housing alternatives are also needed. One key need is information; consumer knowledge about the range of available housing options and sources of payment must increase. Actual assistance and counseling about the most appropriate setting should be available. With the dramatic increase in computer use in the older population, web-based information should be created and promoted. The need for more information and knowledge is not limited to older adults and family members. Community-based service providers also need to have a full understanding of housing options and how housing issues influence other aspects of well-being so appropriate services and referrals can be made.

INDIVIDUAL DIFFERENCES MUST BE RECOGNIZED

One of the strongest findings of the *Pathways* study is that one-size-fits-all solutions are not appropriate. Beyond the original categories of reasons for moving proposed by Litwak and Longino (1987), older persons have a plethora of reasons for considering moving, including the desire to maintain quality of life; the desire to preserve health; the search for more affordable housing; or other, idiosyncratic reasons, ranging from remarriage to a specific leisure-time interest. They also have differing levels of interest in and comfort with the various housing options.

CONSUMER CHOICE AND SOVEREIGNTY SHOULD BE PROMOTED

Underlying this diversity in preferences, however, is the desire of virtually all older adults to be, as much as possible, in control of the housing decisions that determine where they will live. Individuals need to be able to match their needs, personalities, and preferences with a range of settings. They must be given the information to be well-informed consumers of housing and thus be able to choose among existing options. The idea of consumer directed care has gained considerable attention in regard to the type of care older adults receive and who provides it, but the principle has no less applicability to choices of where such care is received.

ENRICHED LIVING ARRANGEMENTS SHOULD BE MADE MORE EASILY AVAILABLE TO LOW-INCOME PEOPLE

The advantages provided by service-rich assisted living, especially in CCRC, should—ideally—be made available to people regardless of income. Given that limited public resources are unlikely to make this possible in the near future, incremental steps would be useful. Greater continuity of care could also be made available to persons with lower incomes through better coordination among existing housing options, especially those intended for this population of seniors. Additionally, creative applications of existing models could increase the types of housing available to those with lower incomes. One example is the "CCRC without walls." Since a large amount of the expense of a CCRC is the bricks and mortar, this model extends the concept of continuing care to those living in their own homes, and it costs much less money than would be required to move to a CCRC (Barbour, 1996). Already in place in a few areas as a private-pay option, public sector incentives and subsidies could help expand its availability.

In conclusion, the findings of the *Pathways* study show clearly that we have a long way to go before these features become established in communities across America, but perhaps not as far as it might seem. To be sure, numerous gaps exist in the housing system described in this volume; inequities exist on the basis of income; and residential moves can at times incur negative consequences. However, it is also clear that numerous options exist, even in a small community, and that areas for improvement can be clearly identified. By acting on such information, we can move toward a more comprehensive system of living arrangements that promotes well-being for older persons.

REFERENCES

Barbour, C.A. (1996). Contining care at home: An innovative alternative to the campus-style continuing care community. *Spectrum, 10*(3), 17–20.

Cohler, B. J. (1983). Autonomy and interdependence in the family of adulthood. *The Gerontologist, 23*, 33–39.

Litwak, E., & Longino, C. F. (1987). Migration patterns among the elderly: A developmental perspective. *The Gerontologist, 27*(3), 266–272.

Luescher, K., & Pillemer, K. (1998). Intergenerational ambivalence: A new approach to the study of parent-child relations in later life. *Journal of Marriage and the Family, 60*, 413–45.

Regnier, V. M. (1994). Assisted-living housing for the elderly: Design innovations from the United States and Europe. New York: Wiley.

CHAPTER 11

Summary and Conclusions

Elaine Wethington and John A. Krout

This chapter synthesizes the findings of the *Pathways to Life Quality* study and provides a comprehensive overview of what we have learned about residential differences and transitions among older people. A special focus of this volume has been to assess the relationship between place of residence and the health and quality of life of older adults. To that end we have looked at variations and changes in social integration, health, utilization of services, stressor exposure, and subjective well-being. We review the implications of our findings for research, theory, and practice as well as discuss the limitations of our findings. We have learned much about the residential diversity and uniqueness of the older people in our study and recommend that future researchers and practitioners incorporate the capacity to allow for diversity in their work with older populations.

MAJOR FINDINGS

In this volume, we address eight major questions:

- What features of senior facilities attract those who plan to relocate?
- What types of changes in health and personal mobility promote residential choice or relocation?
- How do preexisting levels of social integration, support, and health affect the decision to relocate or to age in place?
- Does relocation have an impact on levels of social integration?
- What association does residence have with the use of services?
- Do changes in health and activity over time differ by residential environment?

- How do well-being indicators differ for residents of various living environments?
- What are the implications of our findings for theory, policy, and practice?

WHAT FEATURES OF SENIOR FACILITIES ATTRACT THOSE WHO PLAN TO RELOCATE?

Chapter 2 of this volume examines in detail the reasons older people relocated to new residences. Once the decision to move is made, other factors in the new housing environment begin to become significant. Health is an important reason for moving, regardless of whether *Pathways* respondents were moving to a CCRC or to an independent-living apartment. CCRC residents were interested primarily in the availability of continuing care and on-site medical services. This is a vital consideration for several reasons. Those who move into a CCRC were required to be in fairly good health in order to gain admission. They also had high levels of education, were likely to have anticipated the inevitability of declining health, and as a group had initiated the founding of the facility. Movers to independent-living complexes were in poorer health to begin with and were seeking to remain independent as long as possible. It is likely they waited longer before making the move.

Additionally, maintaining social relationships and connectedness were primary concerns. When asked about the main attractions of the facility, about one third of those moving into a CCRC mentioned living in close proximity to family and friends, living near compatible people, and living close to cultural activities. These movers were seeking to maintain their social ties and previous levels of integration into a familiar community. Similarly, those who moved into an independent-living facility mentioned social relationship and participation as being important considerations in their decisions. Younger respondents and those in better health were more interested in the cultural activities available in their new housing or in the nearby community. It must be noted that more women than men mentioned social relationships and activities as being key reasons for choosing the independent-living apartments.

An important question is whether facilities can be designed to make them more attractive to those who plan to relocate, and more functional and satisfying for those who live in them. In chapter 3, Eshelman, Evans, and Utamura take a unique approach to propose answers to these questions. They examine the relationship between features of community housing and subjective housing satisfaction as reported by members of the community-resident sample in the *Pathways* study. Their findings provide insights into the types of features that promote the personalization of living spaces. Previous work by these researchers has shown that personalization of the living space promotes feelings of well-being (Evans, Kantrowitz, & Eshelman, 2002).

In chapter 3 the authors compare the subjective impact of two types of housing features—those that augment physical functioning for aging people and those that allow residents to personalize their surroundings with objects that provide personal meaning and a sense of home. They found that features that promote meaning are more closely related to housing satisfaction than are features that assist physical functioning. This suggests that managers of facilities should continue to facilitate ways of helping new residents personalize their living spaces.

WHAT TYPES OF CHANGES IN HEALTH AND PERSONAL MOBILITY PROMOTE RESIDENTIAL CHOICE OR RELOCATION?

The design (and timing) of this study gave us the opportunity to interview 101 older people who had their names on a waiting list to move into an independent senior apartment complex that offered some assistance for daily living (meals, housekeeping, social activities, and transportation). At the time of the first interview, these respondents rated the likelihood of moving quite high. However, just one third moved to the facility when it opened. The ones who moved were older, mostly unmarried, and had poorer self-assessed health ratings. However, there were no differences between those who moved and those who did not move in terms of the number of activity limitations they had (Holmes & Wolle, 2001).

During the second interview, we asked the movers why they had decided to move. Their answers indicated a desire for more social interaction as health declined as well as a desire to ease the burden on their families. Typical responses included:

> "I wanted to be around more people and get involved in group activities."
> "I could no longer take care of the house. It was too much for me."
> "I wanted to take the burden off my children. I moved here so they wouldn't worry."

After the second interview, we learned that the majority (74%) of those who were on the waiting list but had not moved had said that they were no longer actively considering a move (Holmes & Wolle, 2001). Thus the decision to relocate is often a dynamic one. We do not yet have a good idea about what types of events or occurrences may divert plans for a move, but we suspect that improved health or informal support from family to help older family members maintain independence may be sufficient causes. However, this does suggest that the decision to move is a complex one, and that the outcome is not clearly determinable from the outset or based on one event.

How do Preexisting Levels of Social Integration, Support, and Health Affect the Decision to Relocate or to Age in Place?

The majority of older adults in our study do not want to move from their homes where they have lived for 20 or more years, on average. They have established relationships with their neighbors, friends, and work colleagues, and often their family are nearby. It can be difficult for seniors to consider moving from what has been familiar for so long.

Previous research by Choi (1996) has shown the majority of older movers report doing so because of health constraints. If current housing limits the ability to live independently, many older people seek an environment that will maximize or extend their ability to do so. Health and mobility factors serve as the primary impetus for moving or for beginning to think about moving. Those who moved to the CCRC desired to remain independent and to spare their families the burden of caregiving. Women who had relocated to the CCRC were concerned about their ability to maintain a home, their ability to get around the community, and their spouses' health. However, for those who moved into independent-living apartments, personal health was a major self-reported reason for moving.

In the *Pathways* study, those in the CCRC not only chose to move there, but planned and coordinated the development of the facility. These residents are highly educated and planned carefully for retirement. They recruited the agency managing the CCRC and subsequently established a resident-run living environment. Many of these older people mentioned their desire to live near people with the same interests and hobbies (Krout, Moen, Holmes, Oggins, & Bowen, 2002). The majority of residents were affiliated with the universities in the area and had established social ties.

The *Pathways* sample also contains a group of randomly selected community residents. Not surprisingly, we found that community-dwelling elders much prefer to age in place in their own homes. They want to keep their homes as they are or make modifications that will enable them to remain there longer (Krout, Holmes, & Wolle, 2000). However, the likelihood that the anticipated aging in place will occur is not related to factors that can be predictive of the likelihood of being able to age in place for a longer time, such as better health, higher income, more neighborhood integration, or greater social support. By continuing to follow these individuals over time, we will gain a better perspective of what enables them to stay in their homes or promotes their moving to a different environment. The critical issue is that there seems to be a substantial misfit between the stated wish to remain in one's home as long as possible and the physical ability to maintain a home without assistance.

DOES RELOCATION HAVE AN IMPACT ON LEVELS OF SOCIAL INTEGRATION?

Section 3 of this volume focuses on the changes in social roles, role identities, social participation, and social integration that aging people experience in a variety of residential settings and in response to relocation. Typically, aging has been viewed as a time of role loss or disengagement, particularly as health declines. Relocation may pose a particular threat to social integration if it leads to the weakening of important personal and community ties. Moen, Dempster-McClain, Erickson, and Boyce address these important issues in chapter 4, examining role participation and role identity over time. They look, in particular, at how specific role changes and relocation affect changes in perceived role identities. The authors demonstrate that role occupation and role identity are separate concepts that must be distinguished from each other in both research and practice. They also show that objective roles and perceived role identities are related, but in complicated ways that are dependent on preexisting health, residential setting, and the type of role being considered.

Social role occupation as well as role identities showed considerable change over time. Residents of the CCRC reported a significant increase in the number of roles occupied between 1998 and 2000. Longer term residents of the CCRC (the founders) who maintained their health were apt to add roles over time, specifically as friend and volunteer. Residents of the CCRC reported a concomitant significant increase in the number of perceived role identities. Thus, in one residential setting in the *Pathways* sample, relocation resulted in increasing role participation for healthy residents. It is important to note, however, that the founders of the CCRC were a special group who helped to plan the facility and established a system of organizations to promote self-governance and encourage social participation and involvement in rewarding activities.

In contrast to the longer term residents of the CCRC, recent movers to any location (between 1998 and 2000) reported occupying significantly fewer roles. The moves themselves were qualitatively different in many ways, with some movers locating within the community and some outside the community, some to independent-living apartments and others to assisted-living residences, and some to service-poor as well as to service-rich settings. The findings do hint that relocation to settings rich in pre-existing organizations that help seniors remain integrated into the community at large or that facilitate continuing role participation have the potential of enhancing social integration. Nevertheless, it is crucial to note that recent movers reported no change in perceived role identities, even though role occupancy declined. An important implication is that a person who no longer occupies a role may continue to maintain the identity of that role and the sense of being engaged in that role. So perceived social integration as well as continued support of role occupancy may be a useful target for intervention by managers of senior housing facilities.

In the subsequent chapter (chapter 5), Erickson and Moen pursue these implications further, considering changes in social integration over time. They consider structural integration (the number of roles that people hold) and psychological integration (the perception of being involved in meaningful social activity) separately. Their findings indicate that recent relocation and residential setting are associated with changes in structural integration and psychological integration across time.

Specifically, they found that increasing functional limitations of members of the *Pathways* sample were associated with declines over time in structural integration, but were not associated with declines in their sense of psychological integration. Being married is associated with greater psychological integration but not with structural integration. Place of residence matters for integration as well. Residents of the CCRC and the independent and assisted-living complex in the sample tended to increase the number of nonfamily roles they occupied. (Indeed, their findings suggest that relocation into an organized senior community may facilitate greater participation in the community.) Yet despite the average increase in the number of nonfamily roles occupied, those who moved to senior housing in the past 5 years tended to show a decrease in their psychological integration, compared to those who remained in the community. For those who relocate (as well as for those who remain in the community), ties with new neighbors, friendships, and religious participation appear to be critical to maintaining a strong sense of psychological integration.

WHAT IS THE ASSOCIATION BETWEEN RESIDENCE AND USE OF SERVICES?

The preceding section focused on the support older people gain from their informal networks. Although it is true that the majority of the support seniors receive is from informal sources, community-based services contribute greatly to the continuing health, productivity, and well-being of older people. Chapter 7, by Holmes, Krout, and Wolle, examines changes in the use of community-based services by *Pathways* community residents and residents in congregate housing facilities. In both wave 1 and wave 2, nearly half of the sample members were making use of community services for older people. Yet in general, service users tended to be unmarried women living in senior housing facilities. Community residents were less likely to use any services (e.g., at wave 2, 33.3% were using at least one service), whereas residents of service-poor facilities were found to be most likely to use community services (68.8% at wave 2). The authors document differences among residence group in the use of specific services, differences that are consistent with the population characteristics of those groups. For example, residents in service-poor housing, who were on average less healthy and more frail, were more likely to use home health care and home-delivered meals. Residents of service-rich facilities, who were living in environments that provide on-site social activities and organizational roles, were less likely to make use of senior centers in the community. (They also had significantly less contact with their children, suggesting that senior housing facilities reduce the need for children to provide assistance and thus relieve older people of feeling that they are "burdens.") Older community members, who were more likely to drive, used significantly less public transportation. Over time, older people in all residential settings increased their use of homemaker assistance, most likely in response to increasing limitations as they age.

DO CHANGES IN HEALTH AND ACTIVITY OVER TIME DIFFER BY RESIDENTIAL ENVIRONMENT?

Respondents in the *Pathways* study live in a variety of residential contexts and we have shown that they bring different health and activity profiles with them to these environments. Although we do not know (yet) how the health and activity profiles change over time for those living in the various environments, we expect to see changes as we continue to follow the samples over time. (The third wave of data collection will enable us to follow their development over 2 more years.)

We do know that residents in the service-poor senior housing environments tend to have a pattern of poorer health behaviors and more serious health conditions, such as heart and lung disease. Additionally, their ability to perform daily activities is much lower than that of their peers in other housing arrangements. Their prospects of living in an independent-living apartment for the long term are not encouraging, particularly if they do not have access to services or the finances to pay for in-home services. Those living in service-rich housing have higher education levels and incomes and tend to report more orthopedic conditions, such as osteoporosis and arthritis. Residents of service-rich housing typically have more activity limitations than those who still reside in their own homes, yet have fewer than those in service-poor housing. However, residents of service-rich facilities participate in a variety of activities, including gardening, golfing, artistic expression, and community events, which to some degree have been enhanced by the organizations active in their facilities as well as by preexisting social contacts among the residents.

Respondents living in the community are in better health and have few activity limitations, as they are younger than the other groups. Many older community residents do not plan to move to any sort of congregate setting in the immediate future, but believe that they might move if their health or the health of their spouses limits their abilities to do what they choose. It is likely that as these people age and their needs change, they will be more likely to consider other housing options. As we have seen with those who reside in senior apartments, options for health care and social activities are expected to influence their final decision.

In addition to the differences documented by Holmes and colleagues in health conditions and activity limitations, Wethington examines changes in perceived health in chapter 8. In community studies, changes in perceived health over time have been shown to predict mortality among older people, over and above changes in physical functioning and the course of disease. People living in service-poor facilities were more likely to show a decline in perceived health between wave 1 and wave 2 than were community residents, which is accounted for by their older age, greater number of health problems, and larger number of chronic financial and other stressors. It is intriguing that residents of the CCRC, despite their advanced age and similar levels of health problems and limitations, were not significantly more likely than community residents to report declining perceived health. This is consistent with the idea that service-rich facilities can help older people maintain their well-being and productivity.

HOW DO WELL-BEING INDICATORS DIFFER FOR RESIDENTS OF VARIOUS LIVING ENVIRONMENTS?

In chapter 9, Boyce, Wethington, and Moen examine changes in psychological well-being across time, utilizing three different measures of well-being. In the so-called paradox of well-being, many older people maintain stable well-being in the face of increasing life events, declining health, and shrinking social networks and resources. The authors find that residents of service-poor senior housing show the most negative profile on multiple measures of psychological well-being. (The analyses of housing satisfaction in chapter 3 suggest that those in service-rich housing would also express greater housing satisfaction because of the greater degree of personalization they could exercise over their larger residences.) However, they do not show significant decreases in well-being between the two waves, indicating that there are important preexisting differences in the well-being of the residential groups that account for the difference. Those who relocated between the two interviews did not show a significant decline in well-being, despite the fact that moving can sometimes be a disruptive event. Residents of service-poor facilities did not show an accelerated decline in well-being; in fact, well-being was remarkably stable.

However, chapter 8 comes to somewhat more pessimistic conclusions about the well-being of those in service-poor facilities, using different indicators of well-being. Perceived physical health can be construed as a measure of well-being as well as a measure of underlying physical health. Similarly, perceived personal mastery of the environment is often viewed as a major component of positive well-being (Ryff & Keyes, 1995). Both perceived physical health and personal mastery declined significantly over time for residents of service-poor facilities in comparison to community residents. Mastery also tended to decline for residents of the CCRC.

WHAT ARE THE IMPLICATIONS OF OUR FINDINGS FOR THEORY, POLICY, AND PRACTICE?

An important goal of this book is to identify and discuss the implications of these researchers' findings for older adults, housing planners, and practitioners. Krout and Pillemer detail many specific implications in chapter 10.

Throughout this study, we have applied the *life course perspective* to achieve greater understanding of the lives of older people across time and how aspects of their lives may vary across residential context. The life course perspective focuses attention on the dynamic process of change and adaptation across the life course as people undergo transitions and weather changing circumstances. Transition is a dynamic process but is dependent on the starting point: People differ in their life trajectories of education, experience, social integration, health, and subjective well-being. These preexisting characteristics play an important role in the way transitions are timed and embraced or resisted. Similarly, the social and physical contexts of the transition matter. The physical environments into which people relocate have impacts on their adaptation to it. The resources available in family networks, residential settings, neighborhoods, and entire communities determine access to resources for coping with aging.

Applying the life course perspective leads researchers and practitioners to consider starting points, continuity or change over time, and the timing of transitions. These points of departure direct attention to the importance of the roles of choice and diversity in the decision-making that is involved in transitions. Relocation in old age must be understood as a process within an individual life's history that reflects the diversity of that person's prior experiences. Housing choice reflects not aging per se but a cumulative set of decisions undertaken within existing financial constraints and personal choices.

One of the most important implications of our findings is that one-size-fits-all solutions applied to senior housing will not work well, given the important individual differences we have found in seniors' backgrounds, life experiences, personality characteristics, social integration, and preferences. Preexisting differences in people are important to understanding the course of health in the later years as well as individuals' adaptation to relocation.

The process of adaptation, moreover, is a dynamic one and older people have the capacity to develop and improve their well-being and productivity. Movers to senior housing facilities should be viewed as having the potential to improve, rather than only to decline. Self-governance and consumer choice must be important components of housing policy.

Another major implication of our study is that the context into which an older person moves is important. Although with only two waves of data we are unable to distinguish between compositional and selection factors that channel people of different capacities into different residential settings, we have learned enough to say that facilities do have the capacity to improve the lives of their residents. Facilities rich in social organizations and links to the community have the potential to help their residents maintain and enhance their levels of social integration and, ultimately, their well-being.

In turn, this suggests that as a society committed to supporting its aging population, we must direct our attention to those who have accumulated economic, social, and physical disadvantages over time. On the one hand, our study has found considerable continuity in well-being and health over time, suggesting that older people are remarkably resilient and maintain their capacity for psychological growth and change. Yet on the other hand, we find that movers to service-poor housing facilities bring with them a complex set of risk factors for aging poorly, including more serious health conditions, lower levels of education and income, poorer health behaviors, fewer social resources, and lower levels of well-being and perceived health. Unfortunately, there is a serious mismatch between the needs of these residents and the resources of their facilities.

The *Pathways* study does suggest many specific ways in which this mismatch could be alleviated. Local hospitals and health agencies could work more closely with senior centers to provide information, education, and referral. Community-based services for older people could target senior housing facilities more directly than they currently do, particularly in rural areas. County-based service providers would benefit from knowing that the needs of residents of senior housing facilities are not always entirely met by those facilities. It is clear that maintaining health and productivity should be a top priority for residents of senior housing facilities. Yet maintaining well-being and social integration is also important, given the relationship of these factors to physical health.

Another major implication of the *Pathways* study is that the needs of movers to senior housing facilities change over time. Planners should develop special programs for recent movers, for whom early intervention might be critical, as well as plan for changes in the needs of the population as it ages in the facility. Recent movers would benefit from knowing that the initial relocation period may be difficult and somewhat isolating. The social dynamics of facilities are often very different from those in the home community. Movers and their families would benefit from programs that are designed to promote their rapid integration into social activities in the facilities, as well as special efforts to help them maintain their pre-existing social contacts.

Educating older people about the benefits and costs of relocating to senior housing should also be a priority. The *Pathways* study suggests that those who plan their moves very deliberately, such as those who moved to the CCRC, reaped the benefits of this planning. Making educational programs and planning services available to those with fewer financial resources should be a policy priority and a social responsibility. Those who develop these programs will need to advertise them widely. As a society, we must also develop social incentives to make use of the planning services available.

CONCLUSION

This book, then, has examined issues that will become even more pivotal as we continue on through the 21st century. What is the optimal time to make a residential move, in terms of both psychological adjustment and health? Which housing arrangement is most conducive to health, life quality, and reduced health care costs? What are the processes through which residential moves are made, and the cost and benefits of not moving? We hope that the findings reported in this book will contribute to our understanding of the answers to these questions. We believe that including variation in residential environments as part of the framework and analysis of longitudinal research can provide needed and unique insights into the quality-of-life status and the changes experienced by older people.

We encourage other researchers to examine the questions identified by the authors of this book. And we suggest that they communicate with housing practitioners on both the design of their research and the meaning and implications of their findings. We also encourage program planners and practitioners to consider the role that residential factors play in the nature and delivery of services that promote the health, independence, and social participation of older adults.

Finally, we urge those engaged in the education of gerontological researchers and practitioners to consider the issues examined in this book. Doing so will surely lead to a better and more comprehensive understanding of aging and how we as professionals and individuals can respond to the needs of an increasingly diverse older population.

REFERENCES

Choi, N. G. (1996). Older persons who move: Reasons and health consequences. *Journal of Applied Gerontology, 15*(3), 325–344.

Evans, G. W., Kantrowitz, E., & Eshelman, P. (2002). Housing quality and psychological well-being among the elderly population. *Journal of Gerontology: Psychological Sciences, 57B*, P381–P383.

Holmes, H. H., & Wolle, S. (2001, May). Anticipated living arrangements of older adults. Paper presented at the annual conference of the Empire State Association of Adult Homes and Assisted Living Facilities, Montreal, Quebec, Canada.

Krout, J. A., Moen, P., Holmes, H. H., Oggins, J., & Bowen, N. (2002). Reasons for relocation to a continuing care retirement community. *Journal of Applied Gerontology, 21*(2), 236–256.

Krout, J. A., Holmes, H. H., & Wolle, S. (2000, November). Anticipated living arrangements of community-dwelling older adults. (*Pathways* Working Paper 00–11). Ithaca, NY: *Pathways to Life Quality* study, Ithaca College and Cornell University.

Ryff, C. D., & Keyes, C. L. M. (1995). The structure of psychological well-being revisited. *Journal of Personality and Social Psychology, 69*(4), 719–727.

Subject Index

Activity limitations
  obesity and, 120
  of *Pathways* respondents, 16–8
  residential environment and, 217–9
  service use and, 145–6
Adult homes, 4
African American, 79
Age
  disability and, 127
  housing satisfaction and, 58
  of *Pathways* respondents, 16–8, 125
  residential relocation and, 38–9
  role occupancy and, 78–9
  service use and, 137–8
  social integration and, 98–9, 106–9
  stress and, 167–71
  well-being and, 183–8
Aging in place, xx, 214–5
  disability and, 132
  environment and, 49
  respondents in the *Pathways* study, 14–5
  services and, 135–6
  stress and, 165–71
  survey results about, 41–2
  trends, 3–4, 33
  well-being and, 183–8, 219
Arthritis, 120, 121, 125, 128

Assisted living facilities, 4
  defined, 4
  in the *Pathways* study, 11
  recommendations about, 206–7
  residential relocation to, 31–2
  services and, 135–6
  stress and, 165–71
  well-being and, 183–91, 219

Baby boomers, xx
Board-and-care homes, 4
Bronfenbrenner Life Course Center, 8

Careers. *See* Employment status
Caregiving
  role occupancy, 104
  trends, 33
  See also Services
Children, adult, relationships with
  residential relocation and, 31–3
  service use and, 145–6
Chores. *See* Homemaker services for seniors
Chronic stressors. *See* Stress
Church attendance. *See* Religious participation
Cohort. *See* Baby boomers
Community-based services. *See* Services